HOME-MADE
HERBAL
COSMETICS

Dr. S. SURESH BABU
M.D. *(Ayurveda)*

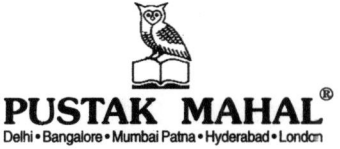

PUSTAK MAHAL®
Delhi • Bangalore • Mumbai Patna • Hyderabad • London

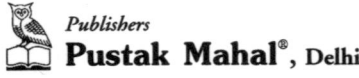

Publishers
Pustak Mahal®, Delhi
J-3/16, Daryaganj, New Delhi-110002
☎ 23276539, 23272783, 23272784 • *Fax:* 011-23260518
E-mail: info@pustakmahal.com • *Website:* www.pustakmahal.com

London Office
5, Roddell Court, Bath Road, Slough SL3OQ J, England
E-mail: pustakmahaluk@pustakmahal.com

Sales Centre
10-B, Netaji Subhash Marg, Daryaganj, New Delhi-110002
☎ 23268292, 23268293, 23279900 • *Fax:* 011-23280567

Branch Offices
Bangalore: ☎ 22234025
E-mail: pmblr@sancharnet.in • pustak@sancharnet.in
Mumbai: ☎ 22010941
E-mail: rapide:t@bom5.vsnl.net.in
Patna: ☎ 3294193 • *Telefax:* 0612-2302719
E-mail: rapidexptn@rediffmail.com
Hyderabad: *Telefax:* 040-24737290
E-mail: pustakmahalhyd@yahoo.co.in

© Pustak Mahal, Delhi

Edition : 2007

ISBN 978-81-223-0775-7

The Copyright of this book, as well as all matter contained herein (including illustrations) rests with the Publishers. No person shall copy the name of the book, its title design, matter and illustrations in any form and in any language, totally or partially or in any distorted form. Anybody doing so shall face legal action and will be responsible for damages.

Printed at : Param Offsetters, Okhla, New Delhi-110020

Dedication
This book is dedicated to my wife Smt. Kalavathi for her all round help throughout my career.
—Dr. S. Suresh Babu

Acknowledgement

I wish to acknowledge Shri Ram Avatar Gupta MD, Pustak Mahal and Shri S.K. Roy (Editor) for the opportunity to write this book. I wish to acknowledge the help rendered by PG Scholars especially Dr. Alivelu Manga, and Dr. Kalyani in collecting the information. I express my special thanks to Dr. Prakash Chandra, reader of the P.G. Unit, for his help with the material.

I am thankful to my son Naveen Shetti, MBA for designing and processing the script, and to Dr. Madhavi Namboodri for correcting the proof carefully.

—Author

Contents

Preface	 6
Introduction	 7
1. Skin Texture	 11
2. Skin Care: The Herbal Way	 14
3. Natural Products & Skin Care	 28
4. Skin Recipes	 35
5. Beauty Foods For The Skin	 47
6. Nail-Care Cosmetics	 53
7. Hand Care	 59
8. Feet Care	 66
9. Hair Care	 73
10. Eye Care	 101
11. Essential Oils	 106
12. Preparing Herbal Cosmetics at Home	 110
13. Aroma Therapy	 121
14. Quick Herbal Remedies	 123
Glossary	..... *125*
Bibliography	..... *127*

Preface

In the 1970s, women used the kitchen as a beauty parlour, as many spices happen to be natural beauty aids. For instance, malai, papaya peel, mashed cucumber, fermented curd, turmeric, lemon etc. are used as herbal cosmetics extensively in beauty care.

Even in the beginning of the 21st century, things have not changed but the style has changed. Now a woman spends about 30 times more money to buy a cucumber face pack or shikakai hair wash.

This purchasing tendency has brought in many herbal cosmetic manufacturers like Shahnaz, Ayur, Pura, Herby, Biotec *et al* into the field and they are not only selling beauty herbs but also dreams. The herbal cosmetic bug had also bitten western celebrities like Barbara Cartland, Princess Diana and Ingrid Bergman. As the demand is going up rapidly, the price of these beauty products is also reaching the sky, leaving the middle-class beauty conscious women and men in a tight corner.

Keeping this in view, the present book *Herbal Cosmetics* is designed and written exclusively for these people, so that they can prepare their own cosmetics with herbs and natural substances available within their reach. All these recipes are well-proven and safe and these are in no way inferior to the market brands and, in fact, are more pure as you yourself are "adding" on genuine ingredients of the recipe.

—*Dr. S. Suresh Babu*

Introduction

Some are born beautiful and others are 'made' beautiful. For both the groups of persons, cosmetics are vital. For the first group of beautiful people, cosmetics are required to maintain their natural beauty and to safeguard from 'environmental hazards', which may affect beauty adversely. For the second category of people, cosmetics are a must to make them attractive. In view of these wider applications, cosmetics are defined as "articles intended to be applied to the human body for cleaning, beautifying or altering the appearance without affecting the body's structure or functions". These articles are primarily of two types:
1. Synthetic Cosmetics.
2. Herbal (Natural) Cosmetics.

The advantages of Herbal Cosmetics are numerous:
1. These, being natural unlike synthetic or chemical substances, do not harm your skin, hair or body and are relatively safe.
2. There is nothing wiser than following one's own tradition and culture. Our culture and traditions are mainly based on Naturals and Herbals.
3. Herbal Cosmetics are in use and practice since thousands of years in India, without any after effects or side effects and are well-proven and documented.
4. The rapid awareness of the bad effects of modern cosmetics prompted a gradual switch-over to herbal cosmetics. The west has turned to the — "Mother-nature-knows-best philosophy" and westerners are turning towards the ancient health traditions of India and China.

This shift in western thought created a giant demand for herbal cosmetics/medications resulting in competition between different players in the cosmetic industry. To mint quick money this unusual rush to produce natural/herbal cosmetics led to a lot of unhealthy competition resulting in adulteration and substitution of costly natural ingredients. The companies producing herbal cosmetics are busy trying to outdo each other through tall, false and unethical claims in the print, TV, Internet and other mass media. Against this backdrop, an attempt has been made in this book to include simple and effective herbal cosmetic recipes which can be prepared fresh at home and used safely without any fear of side effects. These are simple, yet astonishing formulae that suit all segments of people. To illustrate one example, in a recent remarkable study of 50 cases of rough skin due to malnutrition, environmental pollution, chemical cosmetics etc. in the age group of 30 to 50 years, treated with 'Ashwagandha' for 8 weeks, encouraging results were noted. Rough skin became softer; further, the herbs stopped falling of hair in women after delivery. Similarly, many plant remedies make an excellent local application for the infected skin, for instance:

- **Mucilaginous:** Compounds such as those in Aloe-vera (Kumari) are soothing and also provide physical protection and relief from irritation and pain. Further, it ensures faster healing without scars. **Aloe-vera** has rich water holding capacity and works as a good moisturising cream gel.
- **Tannins:** They are present in **Triphala**. They have a pronounced astringent effect and form a tough antiseptic layer over damaged skin tissues. Recommended for the treatment of dandruff.
- **Camphor:** It is an effective antiseptic when used both externally and internally. It is an excellent liniment for skin problems like acne/pimples, apart from its anti-pruritic (itching) action. It gives very good results when used in combination with other herbs. This is why many herbal cosmetics invariably contain camphor as one of the ingredients.
- **Vegetable oils:** They are very nutritive, apart from being useful in burns, scalds and as natural hair oil, e.g. coconut oil.
- **Manjista:** (*Rubia cordifolia*). This is a well-known colouring herb, extensively used as a cosmetic in many products. The colouring matter of the plant is mainly due to the presence of two compounds, purpurins and manjistin. Purpurins are used as deodorant, while manjistin is one of the common ingredients in many hair oils. Manjista acts mainly on skin,

blood and bone tissues, which are vital factors in the maintenance of beauty and youthfulness.

Today, Indian consumers of herbal cosmetic products need not depend solely on traditional Indian herbs, fruits, roots, etc. Many European herbals especially used as cosmetics have made an entry into India. Jojoba, Calendula, Rosemary, Sage, Lavender etc. are examples of this new entry. Therefore, their applications as cosmetics are also included in this work. Galen, a Greek physician, was the first person to create beauty creams by carrying out different experiments in the field of herbal cosmetology. He discovered that vegetable oil could be mixed with water and bees wax to make cold cream, an important base for many herbal cosmetics described in this book. This shows the role of a physician in the research and development of cosmetics, as beauty problems are invariably interlinked with the overall health of the individual consumer and the corrective approach varies from person to person, as "no two persons are alike". This calls for a truly personalised/individual prescription of herbal cosmetics. A viable approach is adopted while enumerating the various cosmetic preparations like creams, oils, lotions, face masks, hair dyes etc. by grouping the consumers in three distinctive categories in accordance with the Ayurvedic philosophy of **Tridosha** i.e. **Vata, Pitta** and **Kapha** types of personality and accordingly a distinct type of herbal cosmetics is recommended to every group of people or consumers. Thus one can prepare the person-specific herbal cosmetics.

Further, it is interesting to note that the analysis of many herbal ingredients using modern scientific technologies has led to the identification of phytochemical components in Indian herbs, which deliver functional benefits like anti-dandruff, deodorant, anti-ageing etc. For almost any European herb containing certain phyto-chemicals, there are Indian alternatives containing identical and similar phytochemicals, For example, witchhazel containing tannins is replicable with ascorbic acid. The ready presence of vitamin C in amla fruit in a stable form enables us to use this amlaki fruit for better anti-wrinkle, anti-oxidant benefits and Sesame oil for vitamin E content etc. In view of the current trend of patenting many Indian herbs the world over, Indian companies dealing with herbal medicines have strengthened their focus on research. This has led to identification of new applications of known herbals. All these inputs made the subject **"Herbal Cosmetics"** richer.

"Beauty is not skin-deep" is quoted often. It is, in true scientific sense, a deep-rooted phenomenon spread over the three VITAL segments of life:

1. EXTERNAL or OUTER Beauty includes the appearance of the skin, hair, nails and teeth.
2. INNER or INTERNAL Beauty is the clarity of mind that oozes personal confidence, while.
3. LASTING Beauty involves the ability to exude radiant health and beauty throughout life.

Health and beauty exist when all physical, mental and emotional components are functioning properly. The herbal approach to health and beauty promotion is typically well suited because it views and treats your problems holistically, balancing well the sensitive mind-body-spirit equilibrium in a natural state wherein we are full of energy, creativity and love. This world's tradition is "beautifully" holistic and accessible to everyone among us. Let us follow the herbal path to be more cheerful, youthful and beautiful.

"There is no cosmetic for beauty, like happiness."
—*Lady Blessington*

Adverse Effects of Modern Cosmetics

⇨ More than 10% of patients examined for contact-allergy, have positive patch tests related to cosmetics.

⇨ The face and the per orbital area are the most frequently affected areas.

⇨ The most often noticed cosmetic sensitizers are fragrances and preservatives.

⇨ Fragrance materials are present in products like perfumes, deodorants, after-shave lotions, cosmetics, toiletries, etc.

⇨ All modern cosmetics contain suitable preservatives to prolong the shelflife of the products.

Source: LA MEDICINE, FRANCE

1. Skin Texture

All of us are born with a gentle, soft and smooth skin, but not many of us can maintain the same texture and tone. This is because most of us deal with our skin carelessly when young, which results in various skin problems affecting beauty. Like any other living tissue, skin too responds to tender care and attention. Therefore, a short review on how the skin functions, is given.

We all begin our lives with a soft and smooth skin, but not many of us can boast of a finely textured skin by the time we are thirty. This is because most of us take our skin, the most widespread part of the body, very much for granted. Remember, your skin can get tired if not looked after and, like any other living tissue, it does respond to tender care and attention. If you realise how full of life your skin is and understand how it functions, skin care will become at once more logical and easy.

Understanding your skin will also enable you to make an active use of your skin in relating more positively to your environment and in communicating with your fellow human beings.

Skin Structure

Skin consists of three layers—the epidermis, the dermis, and the subcutaneous tissue. The surface epidermis is a relatively thin layer; beneath the epidermis is the thicker and much stronger dermis. The subcutaneous tissue or the fat-containing layer lies below the dermis.

The Epidermis

The epidermis is a fairly thin layer. Its thickness varies around the body, depending on the special needs of that area. For instance, the epidermis over the eyelids is particularly thin, while that over the palms and soles is very thick. The epidermis itself is made up of several layers. On the surface is the horny layer—the stratum corneum. This layer is made up of dead cells, which are continuously shed. The cells are shed off as small aggregates, which are normally too small to be seen; sometimes, however, these aggregates become larger and are then visible as scales. This is exactly what happens in dandruff and when our skin is deprived of moisture. Below the layer of dead cells are stacks of living cells comprising the stratum malpighi. This layer produces the main skin protein known as epidermin. The innermost layer of the epidermis is where the new cells are produced. These new cells take about a month to travel to the surface.

In some diseases, however, the movement of the cells to the surface is speeded up and this also results in scaling. The skin pigment, **melanin**, is produced by special cells called melanocytes. Melanin is very important for the protection of the skin from the Sun; this is produced on exposure to the sun, resulting in darkening of the skin.

The Dermis

The dermis is a much thicker layer than the epidermis. It is made up of a connective tissue framework in which are embedded blood vessels, lymph vessels, nerves, several types of glands, hair and a whole variety of cells. The connective tissue of the dermis is made up predominantly of a protein called collagen. Presently, this protein is being popularly used for the treatment of a variety of skin problems like wrinkles and scars. Elastin or elastic fibres are the other type of protein fibres in the dermis. The dermis also contains a complex system of blood and lymph vessels and a highly complicated nervous system. The nerves receive and pass on an endless stream of valuable information to the body. Any type of skin massage is thought to facilitate the drainage of lymph glands and also to enhance the circulation of blood. Similarly, it has been suggested that massage smoothens the nerves in the skin.

According to Ayurveda, **"Bhrajaka pitta"**, a variety of pitta dosha, is responsible for both the constant glow of the skin, which is referred to as **'prabha'** i.e., complexion of the skin, and the quality of blood that is flowing in the deeper layer of the skin.

The Subcutaneous Tissue

Below the dermis is the fat storage area of the skin. The amount of the fat stored varies in different parts of the body. In some parts of the body it has been given fancy names like 'cellulite'. This tissue has been a source of considerable controversy in scientific and cosmetic circles.

The Skin Glands

The dermis has three types of glands: the **Apocrine glands**, the **Eccrine sweat glands**, and the **Sebaceous glands**.

The **apocrine glands** are present in association with the hair follicles. They are found mainly in areas where there is obvious body hair such as in the armpits and around the genital area. These glands are under hormonal control. A large part of the body odour can be traced to the apocrine glands. By themselves, the secretions of these glands are odourless, but bacteria (which are normally present on the skin) act on the secretions to produce the characteristic body odour.

The **eccrine sweat glands** are distributed widely over the skin and produce a much larger amount of secretions. These glands are concerned with the regulation of body temperature. Under normal circumstances, the sweat glands produce about half a litre of sweat in a day. In very hot climates, the secretion of sweat is increased tremendously and as the water is lost, the body cools down.

The **sebaceous glands** are present throughout the entire surface of the skin, except on the palms and soles. They are particularly numerous in the scalp and on the face. These glands open into the hair follicles and secrete an oily lubricant—the sebum. This contains cholesterol, proteins, fatty acids and waxes. Sebum forms a thin film, which lubricates the skin; it also forms a coating on the hairs, keeping them soft and shiny. When sebaceous secretions are inadequate, the epidermis becomes dry and wrinkled and when the glands secrete heavily, the skin becomes oily and shiny.

●●

2. Skin Care: The Herbal Way

The herbal approach of proper skin care is principally based on three essential steps:
- ◆ Cleansing
- ◆ Nourishing
- ◆ Moisturising

Whatever type of skin it is, these three steps are required for external care of the skin to protect it from the constant ill-effects of environment, stress and the skin's natural process of cell degeneration.

Healthy Skin

Normal healthy skin generally has the following features:
- ◆ It is rosy and lustrous.
- ◆ It is unblemished and smooth.
- ◆ It is evenly coloured.
- ◆ It is soft, firm and elastic.

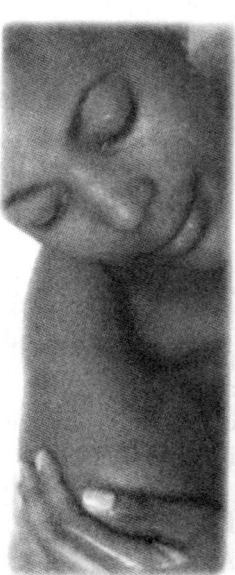

Unhealthy Skin

The unhealthy skin features are:
- ◆ It is dull, sallow and ruddy.
- ◆ It is pale, blemished, dry and discoloured.
- ◆ It is sagging, puffy and wrinkled.

Avoid These Things

- ○ Intake of hot and cold stuff regularly.
- ○ Hot and spicy food.

- Excessive consumption of fish, sour fruits, ice-creams.
- Excessive use of salty items.
- Fried food.
- Junk food.
- Excessive stress.

Drab complexion and lack of glow are the indications of imbalance and premature ageing due to many factors like stress, poor eating habits, improper skin care, exposure to environmental hazards etc. All these unhealthy skin features result from a decline in basic skin functions, such as new cell growth, elastin and collagen production, blood circulation, secretion of ground substances, immune activity and enzyme activity. Therefore, in order to help the skin look young and radiant, our beauty products and treatments must at least provide:

- Exfoliation to remove dead skin cells.
- Epidermal stimulation for new cell growth.
- Anti-oxidant properties for cellular rejuvenation and repair.
- Improved capillary blood flow.
- Immune-stimulation.
- Penetrating moisture and nutrients to replenish all layers of skin tissue.

The three-step process of cleansing, nourishing and moisturing of skin, using only herbs and oils suitable to the individual skin type, fulfils all these basic needs of a healthy and rich skin.

Proper Cleaning

Most herbal systems of medicine like Ayurveda prescribe herbal powders to clean and exfoliate the skin on a daily basis. The herb acts as a gentle scrub to clear away the dirt, toxins, pollutants and dead cells without washing away the necessary moisture ingrained in the skin.

Refreshing, Cleaning Facial

Apply face pack containing turmeric and lime juice regularly. It removes dead skin cells and refreshes the face.

Herbal Cleaning Powders

Skin Type	Herbal Cosmetic	
Vata constitution (dry skin)	Manjista Sariva Triphala Kusta Tulasi Yasti Jeeraka Vacha Tulasi	Preferred Oil Sesame Oil
Pitta constitution (sensitive skin)	Usheera Dhanyaka Daru haridra Chandana Triphala Nimba Mustaka Kamala	Preferred Oil Coconut Oil
Kapha constitution (oily skin)	Lodhra Tulasi Jatiphala Nimba Arjuna Triphala Haridra Mustaka	Preferred Oil Mustard Oil

Triphala

A combination of haritaki, amlaki and vibhitaki in equal ratio alleviates all the *Tridoshas* and maintains the "balanced" state of the skin. Therefore, it can be used in any type of skin.

Gentle Natural Cleansers
1. Milk
2. Sour milk
3. Cream and buttermilk

Proper Nourishing and Moisturising

When the soap bubbles have burst and the skin starts to squeeze, the first thing one looks for after using a harsh cleanser is soothing lotion or cream to replace the natural fluids that were washed away along with the dirt. In Ayurveda, practitioners 'feed' the skin with pure essential oils, which are naturally hydrating and rich in nutrients and also enough to penetrate the skin and rejuvenate the cells. Gentle massage of the skin with the essential oils helps improve blood circulation and strengthen the connective tissue, thereby reducing wrinkles. Further their aroma also helps balance the doshas (vata, pitta, kapha) and the essence itself provides protection from infection.

Since the skin has so many functions and has much to do with the health and beauty of the individual, it should be kept in good form. It should be kept clean not only from outside by frequent cleaning and bathing, but also from inside by avoiding the use of tobacco and other harmful substances, after consumption of which the waste materials have to be excreted by the skin.

General Instructions for Good Skin
Do's

- Wash your skin twice a day, morning and evening, with a soft herbal cleanser and lukewarm water.
- Nourish and moisturise your skin daily with essential oil appropriate for your skin type (please see skin types and suitable oils).
- Avoid excessive exposure to sun, salt-water, wind, cold weather and snow.
- Facial exercise should be done once daily.

Don'ts

- Don't use very oily creams. They clog pores and cause puffiness.
- Don't use soaps or harsh detergents on the face.
- Don't use chemical make-up removers, heavy eye creams or oils. Instead, use cotton dipped in plain vegetable oil to remove eye make-up.
- Don't use harsh scrubs, chemical powders or pumice stones.
- Don't use chemical astringent or products containing alcohol.
- Don't use very hot or very cold water to wash, it breaks capillaries.

- Don't wear make-up when you go to sleep, no matter how tired you are.

Tips for Beautiful Skin in Cold Weather
- According to Ayurveda, cold weather and cool winds, aggravate 'Vata' dosha and cause dry skin conditions, so one has to adjust his lifestyle and diet to add warmth, lubrication and moisture.
- Take fewer baths and showers in the cold season to avoid dryness. When you take a bath, add a few drops of essential oil to the water to provide lubrication. Massage with it before and after showering or bathing.
- Take an occasional steam bath, but avoid saunas, which are dehydrating.

Tips for Beautiful Skin in Hot Weather
- Drink plenty of liquids like water, coconut water, fresh fruit juices, chilled buttermilk etc.
- Keep away from the sun between 11 a.m. and 5 p.m., when it is too hot.
- Use suitable sunscreens, to avoid exposure to the sun, especially if you have sensitive skin.
- Don't drink colas.
- Always use an umbrella in the scorching sun.
- Take bath twice a day with sandalwood or neem-based soaps.

Herbal Cosmetics for Dry Skin (Vata type)
To Cleanse
Preparation

Mix 1 tsp almond powder + ½ tsp dry milk powder + 1 pinch sugar and store in a spice jar.

Application
- In your palm, make a fine paste using ¼ tsp of the above combination with the required quantity of warm water.

- Apply this freshly prepared paste all over the face and neck regions and gently massage it into the skin for about one minute.
- Do not scrub; rinse well with lukewarm water. Do not dry.

To Nourish

Preparation

Mix 10 drops of sesame oil (til oil) with 10 drops of coconut oil + 5 drops each of neem and lemon oil. Store it in a dark glass bottle with a dropper.

Application

Mix 3 drops of nourishing oil (stated above) + 6 drops of pure water in your palm. While your skin is still wet, gently massage this mixture well over the face and neck regions for about one minute or until the skin absorbs all the essential oils.

> Curd is a natural cosmetic for dry skin. Apply fresh curd on face every morning and wash it off after a few minutes with cold water.

To Moisturise

Preparation

Melt ½ oz cocoa butter in a double boiler, add 4 oz avocado or almond oil and remove it from heat. Using a dropper, add 1 oz orange peel oil, one drop at a time, while stirring.

Add 3 or 4 drops each of coconut and rose oil to the mixture when it cools.

- **Weekly Facial Pack**

Apply face pack prepared from honey, curd and egg. Wash it after 30 minutes. This offers nutrition to dry skin.

Application

Apply this freshly prepared moisturising cream gently over the surface of face and neck. Do not massage it into the skin.

Apply as required during the day as per conditions.

- **Natural Face Cream**

Pure honey ½ tsp (5 ml), 'malai' (milk cream) ½ tsp, vegetable oil ½ tsp, glycerin ½ tsp; mix well and apply. Wash off after 30 minutes.

Herbal Cosmetics for Sensitive Skin (Pitta type)

To Cleanse

Preparation

Mix 1 tsp almond oil + ½ tsp orange peel + ½ tsp dry milk, and store the mixture in a spice jar.

Application

- ◆ Make a fine paste by mixing ¼ tsp of the above preparation with required quantity of pure rose water in your palm.
- ◆ Apply this fresh paste all over the face and neck regions and gently massage it into the skin for about one minute.
- ◆ Do not scrub; rinse well with cool water and do not dry.

To Nourish

Preparation

Mix 1 oz almond oil + 10 drops each of rose oil and sandalwood oil.

Mix well and store it in a dark glass bottle with a dropper. It is a good nourishing oil.

Application

In the palm, take 2 to 3 drops of the above nourishing oil and add 4 to 6 drops of water. When your skin is wet, gently massage this mixture all over the face and neck for about one minute.

To Moisturise

Preparation

Melt 1 oz cocoa butter in a double boiler and add 3 oz of sunflower oil. Remove it from stove/heat and then add slowly 2 oz of pure rose water drop by drop, using a clean dropper. Add 5-6 drops of sandalwood oil while stirring the mixture when cool. This is a good moisturiser.

Application

Gently apply this freshly prepared moisturiser over the face and neck; do not massage it into the skin. Apply extra moisturising cream as required.

Herbal Cosmetics for Oily Skin (Kapha type)

To Cleanse

Preparation

- Mix 1 tsp barley meal.
- 1 tsp lemon peel.
- ½ tsp dry milk. Store it in a clean spice jar.
- Powder of orange peel well mixed in water can also be applied 30 minutes before bath. It lightens dark skin.

Application

Make a fine paste in your palm by using ¼ of the above mixture + warm water as required. Apply this paste all over the face and neck and gently massage it into the skin for about a minute. Do not scrub; rinse well with warm water and do not dry.

To Nourish

Preparation

Mix well 1 oz sunflower oil, 10 drops lavender oil, 5 drops bergamot and 5 drops of clay sage oil. Store the mixture in a dark glass bottle with a dropper. It will make a very good nourishing oil.

Application

In the palm of your hand mix 2 drops of the above nourishing oil + 4 drops of pure water. While your skin is still wet, gently massage this mixture all over the face and neck for about one minute.

To Moisturise

Preparation

Melt 1 oz cocoa butter in a double boiler, add 3 oz almond or sunflower oil. Remove it from stove/heat. Using a dropper add 2 oz rose water drop by drop. Add 1 drop of camphor oil + 3 drops of lavender oil while stirring the mixture when cool. It is a good moisturiser.

Application

Gently apply a very small amount of moisturiser over the face and neck; do not massage it into the skin. Use once in the morning and evening only.

Herbal Cosmetics for Combination Skin

If the skin is a combination of dry and oil types, herbals recommended in dry skin are to be used on the areas of dry skin, while herbal cosmetics recommended for oily skin are to be applied on the oily parts of the body.

Herbal Cosmetics for Normal Skin

- This skin is smooth and velvety to touch and does not look puffy.
- It has a rosy colour because of the circulation of blood and the skin is well moisturised.
- The skin pores are fine and barely visible and this type of skin is very rare.

However, though this normal skin is not always problematic, it still requires sensible care and gentle cosmetics of herbal origin. Synthetics can spoil the texture of the skin, *so select cosmetics or skin care products carefully.*

Sun Shields

- Avoid the sun between 11 a.m. and 5 p.m.
- Use a sunscreen with the right sun protection factor (SPF).
- Drink a lot of water and eat a lot of fruits and vegetables.
- Apply two teaspoons of tomato juice and 4 teaspoons of buttermilk, on the face and wash after 30 minutes.
- Mix olive oil with equal quantity of vinegar and apply an hour before you bathe.
- Applying lime and honey is a good practice.
- Always wear a scarf and hat while outdoors.
- In case of sunburn, crush a few fresh strawberries and apply. It is also a popular cosmetic for the complexion and to removes freckles.
- Similarly papaya pulp juice can also be applied on sunburns.

Skin Problem Alert
- When there is discoloration of the skin.
- Excessive dryness of the skin.
- Numbness.
- Lack of sensation.
- Excessive sweating.
- Excessive itching...

...consult your doctor immediately.

Patch Test
Mix one or two drops of essential oil (required) with 1 tsp (5 ml) base oil like coconut oil in a small bowl. Apply this oil on your wrist, inside your upper arm, behind your ear or behind your knee and wait for 12 to 24 hours. If no irritation develops, it is generally safe to use the product.

Certain Practices to Keep Your Skin Glowing

• Exfoliate
Once or twice a week, depending on your skin type, use a gentle combination of natural ingredients to exfoliate or slough off dead skin cells.

The Weekly Fruit Face Mask
Make an exfoliating mask for once-a-week application:
- *DRY SKIN:* Banana or avocado pulp.
- *OILY SKIN:* Strawberry or papaya pulp
- *SENSITIVE SKIN:* Banana or pineapple pulp.
- *COMBINATION SKIN:* Combined approach depending on the combination of skin types of the body, face etc.

'Ahyanga'—The oil bath
A bath after massaging a suitable oil over the entire body, is known as 'Ahyanga' in Ayurvedic parlance. Ahyanga is used to cleanse the body keeping in mind the doshic profile of the skin.

Doshic Profile of Skin

Kapha Prakriti	Pitta Prakriti	Vata Prakriti
Thick, moist, pale	Fair, peachy	Thin, fine-pored
Soft and cool to touch	Soft, lustrous	Cool to touch
Tones well and ages gracefully	Sensitive to touch	Chemically sensitive
Enlarged pores	Oily T-Zone	Dry rashes
Thick oily secretions	Acne, blackheads	Corns and calluses
Dull, sluggish	Rashes, itching	Lack of tone, lustre

- ○ Give a full body massage.
- ○ Increase the heat in your body by exercising.
- ○ Cleanse the body with appropriate herbal powder mixture keeping in mind the "doshic" profile of your skin as given in the table.
- ○ Finally take a warm water bath.

This offers multifaceted benefits like:
- ◆ Slowing down the ageing process.
- ◆ Overcoming fatigue.
- ◆ Controlling body aches.
- ◆ Nourishing the skin and making it soft and silky.
- ◆ Benefiting the eyes.
- ◆ Improving skin resistance.

In short, this weekly oil bath keeps you young, energetic and beautiful.

Different herbs and oils should be used for different skin types.

Dry skin

Such persons should use **sesame oil** enhanced with any one of the following:
- ◆ Aswagandha
- ◆ Shatavari
- ◆ Bala etc.

Sensitive skin
Such persons should use **coconut oil** enhanced with:
- Bhringraj (Ecliptic alba)
- Brahmi
- Chandan (sandalwood).

Oily skin
Such individuals should use **mustard oil** enhanced with:
- Nimba (margoose)
- Jatiphala
- Lodhra etc.

- **Steam Bath**

After cleaning, treat your skin to a steam bath twice or thrice a month to deep-cleanse the pores and stimulate blood circulation. People with oily skin should steam more regularly than those with dry skin.

- **Facial Steam**

To create a facial steam, add 2 to 3 drops of an essential oil that suits your skin type (sandalwood oil is the ideal choice) to a quart-size bowl of steaming hot water. Sit comfortably at a table with the bowl of water in front of you. Be careful not to touch the bowl, lean over it with your face about 10 inches above the water, make a tent with a towel, allowing the steam to caress your face and neck area. Enjoy the relaxing steam treatment for about 10 minutes and treat yourself with a facial mask or toner and moisturiser.

- **Skin Brushing for Better Circulation**

Popular in Northern Europe, skin brushing with a soft, natural-bristle brush is an invigorating way to slough off dead skin and stimulate circulation. You can do it yourself or make it a mutual experience. To brush the skin of your hands, use a light touch and circling movements in a brisk, flicking, upward direction. Begin with brushing the fingers, then move up the hands to the arms, toward the heart. Choose the firmness of the brush according to your skin type. The more fragile your skin, the more gentle the brush.

According to renowned Physiologist Bernell Baldwin, Ph.D., regular daily skin brushing tones the vasomotor, or blood vessel system of the body, making it more efficient.

Caution: Do not practise skin brushing on areas affected by rashes, eczema, or psoriasis. A natural sponge gourd is generally a good choice for skin brushing.

Nutritional Supplements: Synthetic vs. Natural

Unless one eats a 100 percent organic diet, gets all the rest needed, has no stress or strain in life, and lives on a pollution-free planet, one needs some sort of dietary supplement for better health and skin texture. Pesticides, radiation, polluted water, smog, preservatives and antibiotics drain our bodies of essential nutrients. Therefore, one needs a daily supplement. The synthetic or isolated vitamins and minerals, in mega or minute doses, do have their rightful place in the treatment of acute disease or severe nutritional deficiencies.

But for those who are basically healthy and want to use supplements to strengthen the immune system, help prevent disease and improve skin complexion, use of natural, wholefoods and herbs as supplements are the better choice, as these work slowly over a period of time to strengthen the body, add vitality and offer the feeling of well-being, while synthetic vitamins and minerals can produce a drug-like effect. Wholefood means unfractionated, complete and balanced food, just as Mother Nature provides.

> **Share a Secret**
> Eat fruits that are in bright colours like apples, oranges, tomatoes and carrots for glowing skin. This is nature's secret.

Tips:-

- Garlic juice is used as a rubefacient in skin diseases.
- The resin of *Altingia excelsa* (silaras) is useful in affections of skin diseases like scabies and leucoderma.
- *Cocos nucifera* (Nariyal), no doubt its oil is nourishing for hair, it is also useful for ringworm, itch and other skin diseases.

- *Curcuma longa* (haldi) is used in the form of paste with pulp of neem leaves. It can be used on ringworms, itch, eczema and other parasitic skin problems.
- *Ocimum sanctum* (Tulsi) has amazing properties. The juice of the leaves should be taken internally and is very effective in skin diseases such as itches, ringworm and leprosy.

3. Natural Products & Skin Care

Nature has bestowed its enormous wealth on us. We only need to tap the resources. A gateway to health and beauty would open up for us immediately.

Home-made Herbal Cosmetics

Preparation of herbal cosmetics at home is not an impossible task. Beauty consultants make things too complicated. People are made to believe that commercially manufactured cosmetics are better than home-made cosmetics. In fact, they are as good as the commercial products. Since no preservatives are added in them, they have a very short shelf-life. Therefore, they should be prepared in small quantity. However, refrigeration extends their shelf-life for a few more days. Home-made herbal cosmetics have an edge over commercial products since genuine ingredients are mixed in proper proportions which gives authenticity to the products. Creams and emulsions are primarily a mixture of distilled water, oily substances like waxes and fragrance in varying proportions. A slight change in the proportion changes the character of the preparation.

Ayurvedic Herbal Cosmetics

In Ayurveda classics, there are many cosmetic formulations, which are made up of purely herbal and natural substances. These preparations are in use for centuries with a high success rate. Further these can be prepared at home without much difficulty. If one desires, these can be purchased ready-made from any Ayurveda stores. Further to extend shelf-life some preservatives or additives are added.

"Anga Raga Lepa"

"Anga" means body, "Raga" means brightening, and "Lepa" means external application. This includes face brightener. It was formulated by the great Sushruta, the Father of Surgery.

Ingredients

Hareetaki fine powder (harda).
Neem leaves fine powder.
Mango tree bark fine powder.
Dadima flowers powder (dry).
Jasmine leaves powder.

Preparation

Mix all the fine powders in equal quantity and prepare fine paste by adding the required quantity of pure rose water.

Application

Apply this freshly prepared paste on the body, face and neck and massage gently for 10 minutes. Then have lukewarm water bath. Do not use soap regularly. Use this paste in place of soap and see the wonders it works!

Almond Oil

This oil is derived from the ripe, pressed kernel of the fruit. It is edible, non-toxic, and generally very pale yellow in colour.

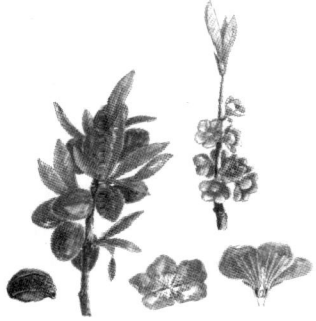

Cosmetic applications

- It is a classic beauty oil that has medium weight and penetrates and pampers the skin wonderfully.
- Almond oil is used in the preparation of beauty creams, lotions, massage oil, lipsticks, and facial cleansers.
- Buy cosmetic grade almond oil and store it in the refrigerator to prevent it from going rancid.

Almond paste/mask for smooth skin

Mix a tablespoonful of almond with enough water to make a paste and rub on the body, skin, face and neck. Leave it on as a mask for above 20 minutes. Rinse off with tepid water. This promotes smoothness of the skin.

Honey

Apart from many medicinal applications, honey has cosmetic value also. That is why honey is an important ingredient of many cosmetic lotions, creams, balms, soaps, facemasks and baths.

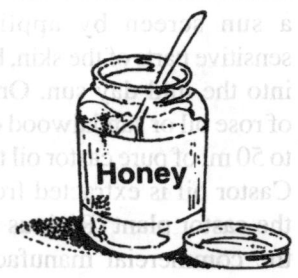

- Honey is a good and gentle antiseptic, highly useful in soft, silky facial skins.
- It's an excellent moisturiser, because of high-content invert sugar.
- It's a good detoxifying gel, makes one's skin radiant by removing environmental toxins accumulated in the skin.
- Regular intake of pure honey provides wholesome nourishment, and is a highly energy-giving food.
- Honey improves the content of RBC and haemoglobin level, because of the presence of iron, magnesium and copper in natural form.
- Beauty depends on good health, more so on good blood circulation. Honey purifies blood and regulates its circulation.

Papaya

Papaya helps in reducing the effect of stress and strain of modern life on the skin. It acts as an exfoliative agent, removes dead cells and peels away dry skin. Raw papaya juice has potent bactericidal properties and is used for many skin infections such as corns, warts and pimples. In skin burn papaya pulp juice is a good natural healing agent.

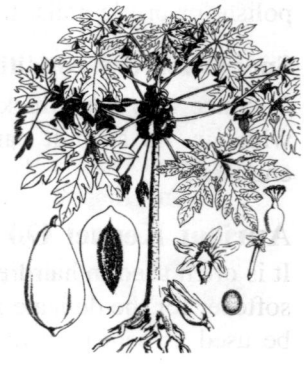

Castor Oil
Herbal sunscreen oil

Castor oil is a rich, smooth oil, which can be used as a protective barrier between the skin and harsh environmental conditions. It can be successfully used as a sun screen by application on the sensitive parts of the skin, before venturing into the mid-day sun. One or two drops of rose oil or sandalwood oil can be added to 50 ml of pure castor oil that is odourless. Castor oil is extracted from the seeds of 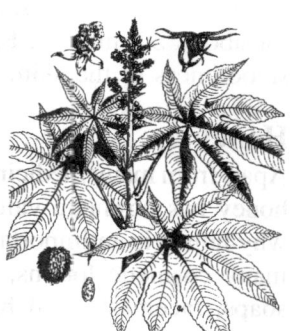 the castor plant (Ricinus communis) and used in vast quantities in the commercial manufacture of lipstick since it is an excellent emollient.

For winter cracked lips

Since castor oil is an excellent emollient, odourless castor oil and sandalwood combination works wonderfully in the condition of cracked lips. In winter, this should be applied regularly to prevent and treat this condition.

As a hair-conditioner

Castor oil and a few drops of jasmine oil becomes an excellent herbal hair conditioner and makes hair shiny.

As a nail polish

Castor oil (odourless variety of Dabur) can be used as nail polish for brittle nails. It offers good results on regular use.

Special for dry conditions

Since it is very thick, this oil dries up on prolonged contact with air. As such it can be used in dry skin as an excellent emollient.

Apricot Kernel Oil for Delicate Skin

It is often used in hairdressing and massage oils. It is an excellent softener for the delicate skin around eyes, mouth and neck. It can be used as cent percent base blend.

Cocoa Butter

It is a wonderful skin lubricant and its natural cocoa scent is acceptable to everyone. Cocoa butter is the solid fat from the roasted-seed of the cocoa plant (Theobroma cocoa), which is composed of 40 to 50 percent solid butter fat. It is solid at room temperature and is a wonderful additive to lotions, creams and soaps, especially if one wants to thicken the texture a bit. If added in a large quantity, cocoa butter may give a slightly yellow tint to many cosmetics and it is used up to 50 percent as a base blend.

Turmeric

The cosmetic value of turmeric probably depends on its bright yellow colour. Curcumin is the chemical that imparts the colour. Turmeric is considered an auspicious cosmetic by the Indian women. Latest research proves its anti-bacterial, anti-allergic, and anti-oxidant effects.

Turmeric/Milk Lotion for Glowing Skin

Preparation

Take ½ teaspoon turmeric powder and mix it with fresh unboiled milk to make a thin and uniform lotion.

Application

Smear the lotion on the face and,
Fumigate with water vapour.
Wash the face with lukewarm water and,
Wipe with smooth linen.

Uses

This practice, when done twice a week, enhances the colour and complexion of the skin. It also prevents black patches on the face.

Nutgrass (Motha/musta)

The roots of the plant have black and aromatic tubers. They are called musta/motha. Because of the specific fragrance it is used as a cosmetic.

Nutgrass (Bath Powder)

Mix 50 grams of nutgrass tubers with 500 grams of whole green gram flour. Mix well and keep in a good plastic container. Prepare paste by adding a little water to 10 grams of the bath powder and rub all over the body just like soap. Wait for 5 to 10 minutes, then rinse away. Avoid soap. This mixture has enough cleansing effects. Regular bath with this powder prevents skin cracks, fungal infections and bad body odour. It also maintains the lustre and smoothness of the skin.

Skin Beauty Through "Panchakarma"

To tackle skin and hair problems like acne, carbuncles, fungal infections, dandruff and falling hair, one needs to develop awareness of the body's systems and cleanse each system. Skin and hair are the barometer of your health. Panchakarma is the therapy of choice in promotion and maintenance of skin beauty as well as hair health. Following are the panchakarma—the five exclusive treatments.

1. Oleation

(Applying purifying oils to the body)

Take a deep permeating massage based on lymphatic drainage systems with sesame, purifying oil made by til and fennel seeds.

2. Purgation

Take a high-fibre diet of bran, muesli, cabbage, apple and guava to cleanse small intestines and reduce excess acid. Take aloe-vera gel mixed with water internally for seven days for easy purgation.

3. Perspiration

After the body massage with til oil, the skin channels open and are ready to expel wastes. Heat and steam open the outer channels and aid the body's natural eliminative process. One-fourth of all waste exits through skin with sweat. Essential oils like thyme and lavender are added to the water in the steam cabinet and the body is allowed to sweat for 15 minutes, with the genital area protected with an undergarment at the time of steaming.

4. Mud-pack treatment

After steaming, a purifying mudpack is made as given below and applied all over the body. You need: one pack sandal face pack, one pack clay mint pack, one special rose pack, one pack spirutone. All packs are mixed together in water and applied all over the body. It is left to oxygenate for 20 minutes, then rinsed off with pure water.

5. Gelation

Once the body is cleansed, it is wiped with a soft muslin cloth and a skin purifying Spirulina gel is applied all over the body and left to dry. Aromatic facial treatment also has this property and is useful for those who are short of time.

Fresh orange juice for glowing skin

The application of fresh orange juice has also been found to be valuable for a glowing complexion. Properly cleaned fingers should be dipped in pure orange juice and applied liberally over face, chin, neck and forehead regularly.

4. Skin Recipes

Herbal Sun Screen

¾ cup (180 ml) hot water, 1 teaspoon (5 ml) lemon juice,
½ teaspoon (2.5 ml) xanthan powder
1 teaspoon (5 ml) castor oil
3 teaspoons (15 ml) hot shear butter or avocado oil
½ teaspoon (50 drops) essential oils or vitamins of your choice (optional)
Titanium dioxide (optional) available from cosmetic supply companies.

Preparation

1. Mix the hot water, lemon juice, and xanthan powder in a kitchen blender.
2. Add the phospholipids and the hot shear butter or avocado oil to the mixture in the blender and blend again for 1 minute.
3. Stir in the essential oils or vitamins if desired.
4. Let it cool to room temperature, and then blend again for 30 seconds.
5. Add titanium dioxide now and blend briefly.
6. Put it into small glasses or plastic jars and keep them overnight. In the morning, you will have an easy, spreadable liposome cream.
7. If you do not add preservatives, you will need to store this cream in the refrigerator.

Application

Smoothen your skin before venturing out into the sun. An outdoor person involved in golf, tennis, gardening, or walking will benefit from a twice-daily application of this moisturising sunscreen. A sun hat, long sleeves shirt and gloves will also help.

For sun protection

Sheared butter has an SPF of 4. However, for greater protection, consider adding titanium dioxide (a natural mineral). For an SPF of 15, add 1½ tablespoons of titanium dioxide. For every 1 unit of SPF that you want to increase, add ½ teaspoon (2.5 ml) more.

Honey Ointment

Take 30 grams of bees wax, 250 ml olive or almond oil, 75 ml honey and 60 drops of desired essential oil like rose oil. Yield makes about a 60 ml jar.

- Melt the wax in butter by stirring well for 10 minutes.
- Add oil to melted wax, stir well until blended.
- Remove from heat, allow it to cool and then add honey. Stir the mixture well.
- Add essential oil (optional).
- Pour it into jars and use smoothly on affected areas.

All-Purpose Face Pack

Take the following powders in given quantities

Sandalwood fine powder 5 grams.

Usheer fine powder 5 grams.

Nagarmotha fine powder 5 grams.

Aswagandha fine powder 5 grams.

Sariba fine powder 5 grams.

Manjista fine powder 5 grams.

Ambehaldi fine powder 5 grams.

Turmeric fine powder 5 grams.

Preparation

Mix it with a pinch of Gairik (red ochre), mix this mixture in milk and multani mitti (as required) and apply it on the face.

Uses

This pack solves all types of skin/cosmetic problems of the face. It is an all-purpose approach.

Maddar (Manjista) Face Paste

Preparation
1. Prepare manjista tea by adding manjista coarse powder to water in 1:4 ratio, and boil till it becomes ¼ of the mixture.
2. Soak 50 grams of lentil (masoor) in the prepared decoction (tea) for 24 hours. Then strain out the decoction.
3. Dry the soaked pulses in the Sun.
4. Make fine powder of the medicated lentil (masoor dal).
5. Mix 1 to 2 teaspoons of powder in rosewater to make thick paste.
6. Apply the paste all over the face, keep for 15 minutes, then wash off with lukewarm water. The face becomes smooth and the complexion improves considerably.

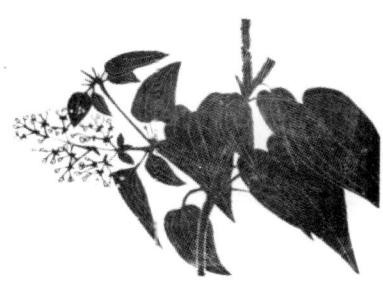

Maddar (Manjista) Body Lotion for Blemish

1. Crush the Indian Maddar roots into coarse powder. Add 3 teaspoons (15 grams) of this powder to 200 ml of water.
2. Boil it on low flame for 12 to 15 minutes and then filter the decoction.
3. Take 10 to 20 ml of decoction and mix it with a teaspoon of honey and stir well to make a uniform lotion.
4. Apply the lotion all over the face, elbows, neck and leave it for about 10 to 15 minutes.
5. Wash the skin with lukewarm water and dry with a soft cotton cloth.

Uses

Using this application twice a week removes and prevents dark spots on the skin as well as darkening beneath the eyes.

Easy Natural Facial Cleaner

This product can be used on any type of skin.

Composition
1. Cosmetic clay—1 tablespoon Kaolin (available at the chemist).
2. Powdered oats—1 tablespoon.
3. Whole milk—2 tablespoons.
4. Lavender essential oil—1 drop.

Method

Mix well all ingredients in a small bowl. Massage evenly and gently over face and neck, using upward, sweeping movements. Rinse well and follow the toner and moisturiser. Any leftover product can be stored in the refrigerator for one or two days.

Saffron for Face Blemish

1. Soak 10 to 20 mg saffron stigma (filaments) in 1 to 2 teaspoons of milk.
2. Stir the milk well.
3. Apply over the face at night.
4. Wash the face with lukewarm water next morning. This saffron mixture keeps the face fresh and smooth especially in winter.

Amla Deodorant Powder

Take dried amla fruit, dried khus grass in equal parts, and grind them into fine powder and add to this green gram flour.

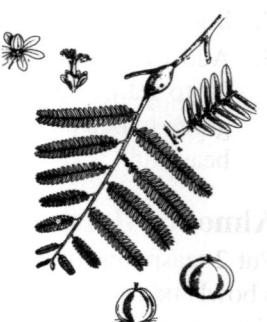

Uses

This powder can be used as bath powder. Add 2 tsp to a bucket full of water, mix well, and use as bath water. It removes bad body odour and brings freshness.

Face Powder—Sandalwood Powder

Take fine sandalwood powder, add 10 grams to 200 grams of plain talcum powder. Mix well and keep for 10-15 days in a clean container. This can be used as a pure cosmetic powder for the face and other delicate parts of the body. It promotes smoothness of the skin and also prevents certain fungal infections in the skin folds.

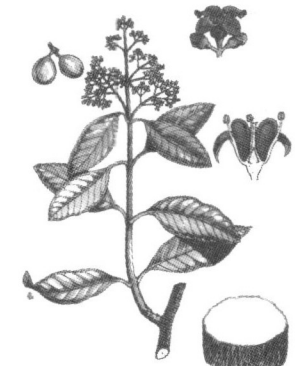

Garlic Oil for Warts

Add freshly peeled and chopped garlic cloves to olive oil.

Preparation
1. Refrigerate the chopped garlic cloves in the oil overnight.
2. Strain out the cloves and pour the oil into a small bottle, with label and date.
3. Store it in the refrigerator.

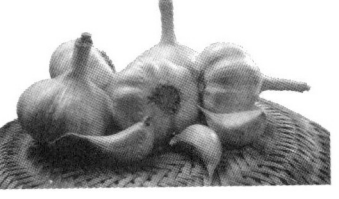

To use
Dab the oil on the wart with a cotton swab or on an adhesive bandage applied to the wart.

Forever Youthful Look

1. Take one glass of boiled milk.
2. Squeeze one full lime and add to the milk.
3. Add 1 teaspoon of vegetable glycerin, stir well and leave it for 20 to 30 minutes, then apply on face, hands and feet before going to bed at night. This makes one look youthful as well as beautiful.

Almond Moisturising Cream

Put 2 teaspoons of beeswax and 1 teaspoon emulsifying wax into a bowl and melt over the water bath. When melted, add 5 teaspoons almond oil. In a separate bowl, heat water to make a common water bath so that the two bowls are at the same temperature. Slowly add water to the melted waxes and oils, stirring all the time. Remove from the heat and continue stirring. When cooled, add a few drops of lavender oil.

Jasmine Moisturising Cream for Greasy Skin

Ingredients

- 2 tablespoons emulsifying wax.
- 2 tablespoons almond or sunflower oil.
- 1 teaspoon lanolin.
- ½ teaspoon borax.
- 1 teaspoon witch-hazel.
- 1½ teaspoons glycerin.
- 8 tablespoons water, and a few drops of jasmine oil.

Melt the wax, oil and lanolin together over a water bath. In a separate bowl heat water, glycerin and borax. Make sure the borax is completely dissolved, and then add witch-hazel. Slowly add water to the oils, and stir constantly until cooled. Then add a few drops of jasmine oil. The non-greasy cream thus formed is very suitable for normal and greasy skins.

Honey Cream

Honey is very useful for dry, coarse and sensitive skin. To make a nourishing honey cream for skin, mix 3 tablespoons of lanolin, ½ tablespoon honey and 1 teaspoon lecithin in a bowl and melt over a water bath. Slowly add 4 tablespoons warm water to it, beating continuously until it cools.

Strawberry Cream for Oily Skin

Put 250 gms of strawberry and 100 gms of sugar in a pan and boil. Cool and boil again. Allow strawberry juice to cool and store in the refrigerator. It is a very useful lotion for oily skin.

Now melt 2 tablespoons each of lanolin and sunflower oil together over a water bath and add the strawberry juice. Remove from heat and stir thoroughly.

Nourishing Cream
Melt the following ingredients together over a water bath:
- 3 tablespoons coconut oil.
- 2 tablespoons olive oil.
- 1 tablespoon almond oil, and
- ½ tablespoon beeswax.

In a separate bowl, dissolve ½ teaspoon borax in 3 tablespoons of heated water. Then slowly add the heated water to oils, and stir until a cool cream is ready.

Acne & Pimple Cream
Preparation

- Neem patra powder (Melia azadirachta) — 3 grams
- Lodhra white powder (Symplocus racermosa) — 1.5 grams
- Harda powder (Curcuma longa)
- Daru haridra powder (Barberis aristata) — 1.2 grams
- Ratanjali powder (Pteris santalinus) — 0.5 grams
- Sukhad powder (Chandan) — 0.5 grams
- Sugandhi khus powder (Andropogon muricatus) — 0.5 grams
- Mulethi powder (Glycyrrhiza glabra) — 0.5 grams
- Manjistha powder (Rubia cordifolia) — 0.5 grams
- Mindhol powder (Randia dumetorum) — 0.25 grams
- Mayu powder (Quercus infectoria) — 0.25 grams
- Vaj powder (Acorus calamus) — 0.10 grams

Applications
Acne, pimples, and other unwanted skin eruptions due to ill treatment of cosmetic origin.

Mode of Application
Take a small quantity of powder, mix it with curd and apply on the face 2-3 times a day.

Acne and Pimple Prevention Cream

For Single Application
- Silk cotton tree thorn powder (Salmalia malabarica) 10 grams.
- Alum powder 2 grams.
- Aloe-vera fresh gel 20 grams.

Mix the ingredients well to a creamy consistency. Apply daily on the face, after a face wash with cold water.

Garlic Night Cream

Preparation

Garlic cloves	20 gm
Vegetable lards	500 gm
Beeswax	15 gm

Put the garlic cloves in a saucepan with vegetable lard and keep it over a low flame for 30 minutes. Turn off the flame, cover the pan and leave it for 5-6 hours. After that remove the garlic cloves and pour the mixtures into screw top jars to solidify. It is very good for sensitive skin.

Apple Night Cream

Preparation

Apple	500 gm (juice)
Vegetable lards	500 gm
Tincture	1 tbsp
Benzoin	
1 cup rose water	

Put the cloves through the blender and add the juice and pulp to vegetable lard. Warm the mixture in a pan over a low flame. Simmer and stir until they get well mixed. Remove from the flame and add tincture of benzoin and rose water. Keep stirring all the time. Strain into a screw-top jar and use as night cream massaging it well on face and neck. It works well for all types of skin.

Almond Night Cream for Dry Skin

Preparation

White wax	30 gm
Almond oil	½ cup
Rose water	¼ cup
Sodium benzoate	½ cup

Melt white wax with almond oil over a very low flame and stir in rose water. When it is cooled add sodium benzoate. Leave it to settle down. After 24 hours it will be a good almond cream to use. It is very effective for dry skin.

Rich Moisturising Lotion

Mix well 100 ml of juice extracted from aloe-vera (kumari) and 100 ml of wheat germ oil. Add some beeswax into it.

Apply over face, and body skin liberally. It is a powerful antioxidant, that tones and softens the skin and prevents skin damage caused by ultraviolet rays and pollution. It is suitable for normal and oily skin.

Moisturising Lotion for Dry and Scaly Skin

Preparation

- Manjista (Rubia cordifolia) decoction 50 ml.
- Aloe-vera juice 50 ml, mix well in a clean bottle and add some cream/beeswax for consistency.

Application

Apply on the skin of the body and face liberally as required.

Benefits

It replenishes the natural moisture of skin lost as a result of exposure to extreme cold temperatures. It also prevents the skin from becoming dry and scaly.

Deep Cleaning Lotion/Facial Cleanser with Toner for All Skin Types

Preparation
- 100 ml of fresh cucumber.
- Soap nut mixed with 10 ml of water.
- Mix them well.

Application
Apply on the face; it is an excellent facial cleanser with toner. It removes dirt and grime and is used as make-up while soothing damaged skin. It keeps facial skin soft and fresh; useful for all skin types.

Gentle Face-Wash Cream

Preparation
Take fresh 20 gm of aloe-vera gel and fresh cucumber juice. Mix them well.

Application
Apply on the face gently. Daily use protects facial skin from dirt, grime and pollutants.

Natural Face-Wash Gel

It is a soap-free herbal recipe and can be used daily.

Preparation
Citrus medica (Bijapura) 20 ml.
Pure honey 50 ml.

Application
Mix well to a gel consistency and apply over the face. Wash off after 20 minutes. It is a natural anti-microbial coolant and antiseptic. It is a daily use face cleanser for oily skin.

Herbal Cold Cream

Preparation
- 4 tablespoons almond oil.
- 1 tablespoon emulsifying wax.
- A little scent and a half cucumber.

Application

Peel half a cucumber and cut it into small pieces. Melt almond oil and emulsifying wax on medium heat and stir simultaneously. When the two get mixed completely, add cucumber pieces. Now heat the contents for one hour on medium heat. Keep stirring simultaneously. Then remove the resultant thick cream from heat. When it cools, fill it in a bottle.

Marigold Cold Cream

Preparation

One can prepare cold cream from marigold petals also. Take about fifty grams fresh marigold petals. Mix them in two litres of water taken in a stainless steel pot. Put the mixture on medium heat, close the lid so that the steam does not escape. Melt emulsifying wax on slow heat in another pot. Now mix the contents of the two and heat it for about fifteen minutes. Let it cool before filling in a bottle.

Nourishing Cream with Cocoa Butter

Preparation

- ◆ 2 tablespoons cocoa butter.
- ◆ 2 tablespoons emulsifying wax.
- ◆ 1 tablespoon beeswax.
- ◆ 4 tablespoons sesame oil.
- ◆ 1 teaspoon almond oil.

Application

Put all these ingredients together on medium heat and stir. When the mixture melts, remove it from heat but keep stirring till it cools. While it is cooling, add a few drops of perfume. When a thick paste emerges, store it in a bottle.

Protective Lip Salve

Protective lip softener prevents chapping, drying and cracking of the lips.

Preparation

- ◆ Fresh juice of carrot 10 ml.

- Wheat germ oil, beeswax 15 ml as required.

Application

Mix them well and apply. It is suitable for all skin types.

Baby Herbal Cosmetics

1. Baby powder

- 5-10 drops of lavender.
- 2-3 drops cornstarch.

Note: When mixing a fine powder like cornstarch with oil, it can be a very messy proposition. The best method for accomplishing this is to mix the components in a plastic sandwich bag, work out the clumps, and you'll end up with a smooth, scented powder.

2. Baby oil for tender skin

- 5-10 drops lavender.
- 2-3 tablespoons olive oil (or any other carrier oil).
- 30-40 drops essential oil.
- 2-3 tablespoons cornstarch.
- Apply all over the body, before taking bath everyday.

5. Beauty Foods For The Skin

Camphor, sulphur, onion, garlic, curd, yeast, Fuller's earth, herbs and vegetable juices are all useful in treating a blemished pimply skin. Here are a few recipes (masks), which are beneficial for such types of skin.

Camphor Mask
Camphor BP has a healing, soothing and tightening effect on the skin. Mix together ½ teaspoon oatmeal, ½ teaspoon camphor BP crystals (or three drops of camphor spirit) and 1 teaspoon orange-flower water. Apply and leave on for 15 to 20 minutes and wash off with lukewarm water. Two drops of camphor spirit when mixed with one tablespoon tomato juice and 1 teaspoon honey, makes a strong astringent skin tonic. This tonic should be left on the skin for about 15 minutes. To improve your skin and cure spots apply the following home-made skin tonic. Put 1 tablespoon glycerin, ½ tablespoon borax powder, 1 cup distilled water and 3 drops camphor spirit in a large bottle and shake well.

Onion Kaolin Mask
Mash and sieve the onion, and mix onion juice into paste with 1 tablespoon of Fuller's earth or Kaolin and 1 teaspoon of honey. It is good to prevent blemishes and wrinkles.

Garlic-Egg White Mask
Beat one egg white, and then add to it the following ingredients to make a paste:
- 1 teaspoon Kaolin.
- 1 teaspoon honey.
- 1 teaspoon carrot juice, and
- 1 clove of garlic.

    It prevents wrinkles and blemishes from your face.

Egg White Mask

Beat one egg white and spread a thin film on your face. Rinse off after 10 to 20 minutes. The mask tightens up the skin and irons out wrinkles.

Anti-Wrinkle Gel

Apply a face pack made up of egg yolk 1 tsp and pure honey 2 tsp once a day and see the wonders!

It removes wrinkles.

Orange Flower Anti-Wrinkle Cream

Ingredients

- 2 teaspoons beeswax.
- 2 teaspoons emulsifying wax.
- 8 teaspoons almond oil.
- 4 teaspoons lanolin.
- 4 teaspoons coconut oil.
- 6 teaspoons orange flower water, and a few drops of tincture of benzoin and orange oil.

Melt the waxes and oils together and add the heated orange flower and drops of tincture of benzoin and orange oil to it, stirring continuously. Besides nourishing, this cream helps to clear lines and wrinkles.

Anti-Wrinkle Cream

It is a facial cream to prevent premature ageing of skin. Regular application delays wrinkles and smoothens fine lines. This contains natural alpha hydroxyl acids (AHAs), skin nutrients and vitamins.

Preparation

- Vitis vinifera (grapes) 10 ml (2 tsp).
- Citrus lemon 5 ml (1 tsp).
- Solanum lycopersicum (tomato) 20 ml (4 tsp).
- Aloe-vera fresh gel 50 ml (10 tsp).

Application

Mix well to a cream-like consistency and apply over the skin daily to prevent wrinkle formation.

Mint Anti-wrinkle Lotion

Mix the following ingredients and use as an anti-wrinkle lotion:
- 2 tablespoons cucumber/mint mixture.
- 4 drops peppermint extract, and a pinch of alum powder.

This lotion can be stored in the refrigerator for a long time. Here is another type of mint mask, which is quite suitable for oily skins. Mix the egg white (of one egg) and 1 teaspoon Kaolin together into a paste and add ¼ teaspoon peppermint extract (or oil). It is good to tighten and stimulate the skin.

Camphor Astringent After Shave Lotion

Mix together in a large bottle ½ cup rose water, ½ cup witch-hazel, and ½ cup distilled water, 1 tablespoon camphor spirit and 2 drops blue colouring. To make the astringent stronger add a pinch of alum. Strain and use to tighten and tone the skin. This recipe is especially useful if you suffer from large pores and spots. Men can also use it as an after-shave lotion. A well-balanced diet, scrupulous cleanliness and skin care, regular elimination, fresh air and exercise are sufficient for a lovely skin. Ancient women used to rub breadcrumbs soaked in milk and honey on their face, and leave it overnight. Pears contain a disinfectant and have an astringent action on the skin. Mash ripe pears, sieve it and use it as it is or mix it into a paste with powdered milk. This recipe is especially good for use on greasy, spotty skins. Here is another bleaching mask especially good for a discoloured neck. Mix the following ingredients together into a paste and apply for 20 to 30 minutes.

- 2 tablespoons ordinary Fuller's earth.
- 2 tablespoons ordinary milk or whey (watery part of curd).
- 1 tablespoon orange flower water.
- 1 tablespoon honey.
- A pinch of ground clove, and
- A pinch of bicarbonate of soda.

This mask tightens and bleaches the skin, and leaves it feeling smooth and fresh.

Egg and Yeast Mask

Mix together egg yolk, 1 tablespoon brewers' yeast and 1 teaspoon sunflower oil into a paste and apply. Leave it on for 15 minutes and rinse it off with milk. This is especially good for a spotty skin.

Almond Mask

Mix together 2 teaspoons ground almonds, 1 teaspoon rose water and ½ teaspoon honey into a paste and apply on the face. Leave it on for 15 minutes, and then rinse off with rose water.

Face Flower Mask

- Flower (Sambucus nigra) – 50g
- Plain Curd – 150g

Prepare paste of flower. Add curd to this and mix thoroughly and apply properly to the face.

Massage it well and leave for about 20 minutes then rinse it off with cold water. The mildly astringent action of the flower helps smooth the skin, bleach freckles and relieve sunburn.

Oil and Tea Cream for Sunburn

No doubt vitamin D produced by sun rays is necessary for healthy bones, but the worst thing we could do for our skin is to expose it to the sun. The sun's reaction on the skin is similar to that of age. It dehydrates the skin leaving it thick, leathery, wrinkled, patchy and dry. It is advised to drink three to four glasses of limewater before going out in the sun. There are several easy-to-make suntan lotions and creams to face ultraviolet rays.

Preparation

- 4 tablespoons lanolin.
- 3 tablespoons sesame oil.
- 2 tablespoons almond oil.
- ½ cup strong tea, and
- Perfume.

Make strong tea, remove from heat and strain. Melt oils in an enamel bowl over a water bath. Now slowly add the tea and beat continuously with a wooden spoon. Add perfume when it is cool.

Lanolin and almond oil keep the skin moist while sesame oil has the properties to absorb ultraviolet rays. The tannin available in tea also absorbs the sun's burning rays.

Nature's Herbs

There are certain medicinal plants, which have been used for centuries in India for enhancing beauty. But to obtain maximum benefits, the use of these plants has to be coupled with the dietary and lifestyle changes discussed earlier.

- Arjun (Terminalia arjuna)—the bark has healing and anti-inflammatory actions.
- Neem (Adirachta indica)—it is useful in many skin disorders.
- Chandan (Santalam alba)—stem powder or sandalwood oil helps in itching and burning sensation of the skin. By its anti-inflammatory action, it is useful in acne.
- Khadir (Acacia catechu)—its bark acts as a blood purifier; hence it is used orally in skin disorders.
- Kumari (Aloe-vera)—gel obtained from the leaves acts on many systems in the body. Regular consumption of gel delays ageing of skin and hair and acts as a rejuvenator. The gel is applied locally on the face for removing scars. It has a soothing effect.
- Manjista (Rubia cordifolia)—local application of the root powder is effective in acne, heals scars and enhances complexion. It is also taken orally in the form of Manjista kadha or Manjistadi churan.
- Yashtimadhu (Glycyrrhiza glabra)—it relieves pain and burning and has anti-inflammatory action. It effectively enhances complexion.
- Haridra (Curcuma longa)—a herb that is well known for its anti-inflammatory, blood purification and wound-healing properties. It also enhances complexion, if taken orally.
- Shalmali (Salmalis malabarica)—powdered thorn of this tree is used for local application on the face for relieving black spots and acne.

- Eraandkarkati (Carica papaya)—the pulp of the fruit is good nutrition for the skin. Its local application on the face is useful in acne, black spots and scars.
- Panchavalkal—this is a powdered mixture of barks of five different trees. It has anti-inflammatory and wound healing actions. Locally, it cures acne and helps in scar healing.

Ayurveda suggests a total skin care regimen considering skin care and lifestyle changes along with medicines. If one follows these principles in diet and lifestyle, then a healthy skin is always within reach. If one does not follow them, skin diseases are likely to occur. Though Ayurveda also has a lot to offer in the area of skin diseases, the age-old saying stands true: 'Prevention is better than cure!'

Anti-wrinkle properties of Aloe-vera

- Greek and Egyptian women in the court of Alexander the Great used Aloe as a natural cosmetic to clean skin of blemishes and glow new and healthy tissues.
- In the USA Aloe gel is used in making a wide range of cosmetics such as sun-tan lotions, face creams, cleaning creams, rouge and lipsticks.
- Use of gel is used remove ageing lines of the face and throat.
- Aloe is used as an after shave lotion which is found to very good and helps to glow skin instantly.
- The pulp is blended into an egg-white to make gel. Two parts of gel blended with one part of base may be used as a face wash to remove wrinkles.
- Dissolved in spirit it is used as a hair dye.
- Application of Aloe gel on scalp will make up the dormant cells. It is a boon for baldness.

••

6. Nail-Care Cosmetics

Healthy nails are a sign of general good health. Chapped or broken nails indicate nutritional deficiency and lack of care. Nail care is very important to maintain healthy profile.

Amazing Aloe-vera

According to legend, aloe grew in the Garden of Eden. This is succulent, native to Africa, has a traditional use for healing wounds and as an anti-fungal agent. A multifunctional plant used for a wide range of basic first-aid purposes, its leaf produces a gel that is helpful 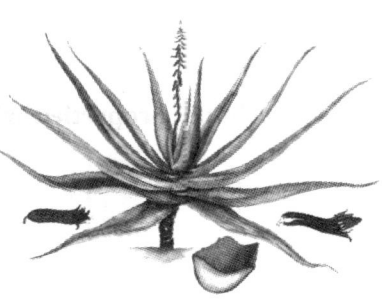 for treating sunburn, wrinkles, insect bites, skin irritations, scarring, and minor cuts and scratches. To cultivate aloe, plant in full sun. Water regularly, but allow the soil to dry out between watering. In temperate climates, you can grow aloe in a sunny window.

Nail-biting Preventive

A worthy alternative to the chemical polish product is a natural ointment made from the gel of fresh aloe-vera leaves.

Preparation

1. Cut a fresh leaf down the centre. With a spoon, scoop out the gel.
2. When you have collected a quantity of gel, place it in a double boiler.
3. Boil the "sticky stuff" down to a thicker paste-like consistency.
4. Store in a small clean jar with lid. Label, date, and store it in a cool place.

Application
When the urge arises to nibble on your fingernails, rub the aloe paste on the edges of the nails. The taste should discourage you.

Caution
A little bit of this gel goes a long way. Large internal doses of concentrated aloe can cause vomiting. A pregnant woman might be tempted to nibble despite the application of ointment, in which case, avoid this remedy, as the plant's anthraquinone glycosides are purgative.

For Infected Nails
Try a warm compress of fresh aloe-vera gel. Squeeze the gel directly on the infected finger and cover with a warm, slightly damp cotton cloth.

Caring for your Hangnails
Hangnails, fleshy bits of dry skin that have split away from the edges of the fingernail, are very common in nail-biters. They can be painful and become a site for secondary infections. Children often have hangnails. This is a good time to give them some direction on how to keep their skin and nails fit. Suggest that they resist the temptation to tear off a hangnail. If it is in the way, cut the flap of skin at its base with clippers or small scissors. Store a bottle or tube of hand cream at every sink and try to get the family in the habit of using it after hand washing. Hangnails can also signal dry cuticles caused by frequent hand washing, cold weather, or rough working conditions. Moisturise the nails and skin around them often. Regularly moisturising the cuticle area will help cut down on the urge to bite.

Protecting Nail Infections
When you have an infection around your nails, wear protective gloves to do wet work on such tasks as washing dishes, cars, laundry, and gardening. Turn the gloves inside out and wash them at least once a week. When the infection is gone, toss the gloves.

Lemon Folk Remedy

In addition to relieving the pain of infection, this treatment will remove stains from your nails. A bonus is that lemon juice restores the natural pH of your skin.

Take 1 or 2 lemons.

Cut a small opening at the end of a lemon and push in the affected finger.

Keep the infected finger in place until the lemon ceases to draw (stops stinging). If you wish, apply another lemon until the pain is relieved.

Note: If the infection or inflammation continues for a time, the nail will lose lustre and have ridges, and the developing nail will be affected. When home remedies do not work, it's time to consult a dermatologist who specialises in nail problems.

Thuja: A Homeopathic Remedy

A homeopathic remedy for brittle nails is Thuja 6x. You should be able to obtain this treatment in stores selling medicinal herbs or from a homeopathic specialist. Thuja 6x is made from the fresh, green twigs of the American arborvitae or Eastern white cedar. These branches contain thujone—a volatile oil that is said to affect the concentration of salt, water, and electrolytes in the body—as well as other wax, resin, and gelatinous ingredients. It encourages moisturisation and helps prevent and heal brittle or split nails. Thuja is best in a homeopathic, diluted dose because it can be toxic when taken at full strength and in excess.

Caution

Pregnant women and people with irritant, dry coughs should not take thuja.

Mehndi: Body Art with Henna

Mehndi is the 5000-year-old traditional art of adorning the fingers, hands, forearms, toes, and shins with a non-permanent dye paste made from the leaves of the henna plant. Hand and body henna designs vary from large floral patterns in Arab countries to fine, lacy paisleys in India to bold geometric patterns in Africa. Henna designs will usually last for 4 to 6 weeks.

Painting with henna is more than a decorative art. In some countries people believe it has healing properties, and it is used in place of gloves; in others, there is a mystical, protective connotation allied with its use, especially in marriage rituals.

Henna Nail Paste

Henna has wonderful conditioning and nail-strengthening properties. This is a fun natural nail treatment with children or on your own.

Preparation

Add the henna to warm, boiled water and mix well, using a non-metal stirring spoon.

½ cup (125 ml) boiled water.
½ teaspoon (2.5 ml) uncoloured, natural henna powder.

Make a paste of the mixture and place it in a small jar with a screw-top lid.

Application

Using a chapstick, glob the henna paste on each of your clean, dry nails.

Let the henna paste dry on your nails and cuticles for 10 minutes. You will feel a pleasant "drawing" sensation. Afterwards, rinse your fingers, towel dry, and gently buff the nails. You can use natural henna once or twice a week for nail conditioning. Remember to stir the henna mixture each time.

Almond Joy

Eat 6 raw almonds everyday to relieve splitting of the fingernails. Linoleic acid, an essential fatty acid (EFA), is one of the important components of almonds. Among other benefits, EFAs help lubricate the body's cells.

The Birth of Nail Polish

You can thank Henry Ford and his automobiles for the development of nail polish. After World War I, there was a large supply of leftover nitrocellulose, which had been used for military explosives. By trial and error, a brave soldier experimenting with the material discovered that boiling the nitrocellulose causes it to become soluble in organic solvents. When these solvents evaporate, the resulting material is a glossy, hard lacquer.

Around 1920, the automobile industry became interested in developing this unique lacquer process for painting new, assembly-line cars. Nitrocellulose lacquer was the paint of choice for Fords. Not long afterward, the beauty industry refined the lacquer formula by adding softening resins as the basis for nail polish.

Allergy to Nail Polish

Allergic reactions to nail polish may surface first on your eyelids; if after applying a new nail polish your eyelids become red and swollen, this is your clue. Because eyelid skin is so delicate, it is particularly susceptible to contact dermatitis. (This means your nails or hands have rubbed your eyes.)

Natural Home Manicure

Taking care of your hard-working nails can be a relaxing, pleasant experience. Plan now to treat yourself to a scheduled home manicure every two weeks, and allow time for between manicure touch-ups and nail maintenance as needed. (However, if a do-it-yourself manicure is not for you, you might still want to read through the following step-by-step instructions—they will help you decide the extent of a manicure you may want from a salon, as well as evaluate their techniques.) When done with a little care, a manicure will offer protection for your nails by eliminating rough edges, coating the nail surface, and helping to improve your self-image. Put on your favourite music. Cut some flowers from the garden or buy a bouquet. Take a lazy bath and set the mood for feeling good before you begin your manicure.

Manicures were first introduced in the United States of America in barber shops. The original barber chair was built with a hollow in each armrest with bowls for hand soaking. During a routine haircut and shave, customers primed their nails for manicures.

Pineapple-Yoghurt Nailsoak

Patricia Rivers-Sergienko, a natural nail care professional, shares this recipe. Pineapple contains two helpful ingredients: bromelain, an enzyme that can reduce inflammation and pain, and alpha-hydroxyl acids, which peel off dead skin cells. Yoghurt is very nourishing and a natural healer.

Composition
- ½ teaspoon (2.5 ml) apple cider vinegar.
- 1 tablespoon (5 ml) olive oil.
- 2 tablespoons (30 ml) pineapple juice, fresh or canned.
- 2 tablespoons (30 ml) plain organic yoghurt, regular or nonfat.

Preparation
1. Measure each ingredient and add to a bowl.
2. Whip mixture with a fork until it becomes blended and creamy.

Application
1. Dip fingers in the bowl and relax, allowing each hand to sit in the mixture for 5 minutes.
2. Massage both hands and fingers with the pineapple-yoghurt mixture. Leave on skin for a few more minutes. Then rinse in warm water and pat dry. Use a fresh batch each time you do a manicure.

To destroy Nail Fungus

Nail fungus is very common complaint of people especially women and mostly in feet. It can be easily get rid of by using/applying paste of Henna continuously for a fortnight at the time of one going to bed. It can be washed next morning but avoid to put your feet into water too much.

●●

7. Hand Care

Human skin comes wrapped and sealed with its own natural skin cream made of sebum, lecithin, cholesterol, and water. We do the best to break down this natural environmental barrier using hot water, detergents, solvents, polishes, and waxes that dehydrate the skin and remove its natural protective oils.

Protective Gloves

We have such a compulsion to keep things clean and shiny that it is difficult to keep our naked hands out of hot water. This behaviour often results in **"dishpan hands"** and yeast infections around the nails. In solving this dilemma, gloves come to the rescue. Whether you are washing, cleaning, or otherwise handling harsh materials, wear water gloves to protect your hands against the elements. Fabrics for gloves have come a long way from the days of metal chains, linen, and silk. Today gloves and mittens are made from every material you can think of, including canvas, cotton, nylon, terrycot, wool, cowhide, deerskin, goatskin, latex, pigskin, and polypropylene, rubber, suede, split leather, and vinyl. Gloves are also available in every colour of the rainbow and more. There are camouflage gloves for sportsmen; garden gloves with floral prints; water-repellent gloves with cotton-knit lining in colours coordinated to match any kitchen; and fluorescent, neon gloves with foam insulation and fleece lining ideal for shovelling snow while also making the occasional lost glove visible in a snowy yard.

There are varieties of gloves available today for every purpose you can imagine, and even for some you never imagined. In many cases, each glove is designed and manufactured to protect the hand against a particular environmental, chemical, or skin-destructive condition.

Natural and Herbal Hand Cleansers

Milky way

Milk, sour milk, cream and buttermilk are all gentle skin cleansers. The next time you're in the kitchen, try washing with ¼ cup (60 ml) of fresh or sour milk, buttermilk or cream instead of one of the liquid dish detergents. It is a surprisingly pleasant experience. To remove greasy substances not removed by water or milk, try an exfoliate such as cornmeal or oatmeal. A heavy hand is not needed. The grainy texture releases both dirt and dead surface skin while stimulating the new skin cells below.

Grimy Hands Soap Substitute

Make a batch to have "on hand".

Composition

- 1 cup (250 ml) cornmeal or oatmeal finely ground.
- 2 cups (500 ml) white kaolin clay, finely powdered.
- ¼ cup (60 ml) almonds finely ground (leave just a bit of grittiness).
- $1/_8$ cup (30 ml) dried lavender blossoms, finely powdered.
- $1/_8$ cup (30 ml) dried rose petals, finely powdered.
- Little drops of the essential oil of your choice (optional).
- A pinch powdered vitamin C (optional).
- Liquid contents of a 400 IU vitamin E capsule (optional).

Preparation

Stir all ingredients together in a bowl and pour into a large jar. Store jar in a dry, cool location.

Application

1. Mix 1 or 2 teaspoons (5-10 ml) of the cleansing grains with water.
2. Stir into a paste by rubbing your hands in a circular motion. Then work the grains up each individual finger and over the back of the hand.
3. Rinse with cool or lukewarm water. Pat dry.

Caution

This recipe may irritate cut or bothered skin.

Lemonade Hands

This is a simple recipe that offers great results in improving the texture of your skin.

Composition
- 1 tablespoon (15 ml) granulated sugar.
- Fresh lemon juice to make a paste.

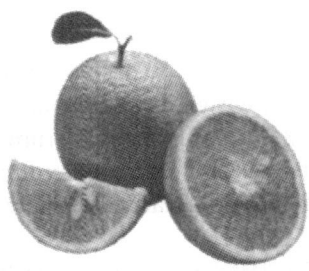

Preparation
1. Pour about 1 tablespoon of granulated sugar in the palm of your hand.
2. Squeeze enough juice from a fresh lemon wedge to make a paste.

Application
1. Rub your hands together in a rotary motion, either clockwise or anti-clockwise. At first, the sensation will be one of a gritty surface.
2. Continue rubbing. The heat of your hands will melt the sugar to become a candy glaze.
3. Work this glaze up and over each finger and over the back of each hand.
4. Leave the glaze on your hands for 5 minutes.
5. Rinse with warm water. Pat your hands totally dry with a soft paper towel.

Natural and Herbal Hand Creams

If you want smoother skin, get in the habit of using protective hand and nail creams. These creams help the skin retain moisture by adding to the natural, water-resistant (lipid) barrier between you and the environment. Soaps and detergents constantly erode this barrier. When applied to slightly damp skin, emollient creams, lotions, and ointments slowly evaporate and hold on to vital moisture. Which moisturisers are the best? The choice is yours. You might decide that at work you want a hand emollient that dries quickly and has no fragrance, has an oil-in-water (O/W) base, and is lotion formula. At home you may use a water-in-oil (W/O) base, a cream formula, and one that you can wear all night with cotton gloves.

Hand Smooth Lotion

Composition
- 1 tablespoon (15 ml) glycerin.
- 1 tablespoon (15 ml) rose water.
- 1 tablespoon (15 ml) Manjista (Maddar) extract.
- 3 tablespoons (45 ml) honey.

Preparation
1. Blend all the ingredients in a bottle and shake well.
2. Store in the refrigerator.

Application
Pour a small amount into the palm of your hands and gently massage onto your hands and fingers.

Cool Potato Burn Relief

A burn pulls moisture from the skin. Applying fresh slices of potato to the burn is very cooling, and the skin will "drink" in the moisture.

Preparation
Peel a raw potato and cut it into thin slices, or pulp it with a hand grater or food processor.

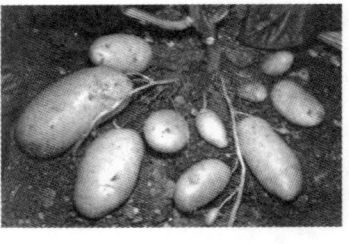

Application
1. Apply the potato slices or raw pulp to soothe minor burns, an itchy rash, or bruises.
2. Apply fresh slices or pulp as each becomes dry.

Special Wash for Chapped Hands

This is a gentle cleanser that is not irritating to the skin. If you repeat this regimen day and night several times a week, your chapped hands will become a thing of the past. (The cornmeal accomplishes by a gentle abrasive action what a harsh soap does by chemical action. The cornmeal, however, does not draw all the moisture away from the important lower layers of the skin.).

Preparation
1. Peel the cucumber and remove the seeds; blend or juice the vegetable for a few seconds. Mix with the honey and set aside in a small bowl.
2. Make a cornmeal paste by mixing warm water, soap, and cornmeal.

Application
1. Wash your hands thoroughly with the cornmeal paste. Then rinse hands well in clean, warm (not hot) water. This helps to remove flaking skin cells and any soluble environmental pollutants.
2. While your hands are damp, apply the cucumber juice and honey mixture. Have someone help you wrap your hands in plastic wrap or insert them in large, zip-seal plastic bags. Cover with a towel, and then relax as long as possible.
3. Rinse and dry hands. Apply moisture cream. If you've done this at night, wear loose-fitting cotton gloves to bed. (Wash the gloves regularly).
4. Repeat this cornmeal wash daily (and repeat as often as you can for badly chapped hands). In cold weather, substitute a cold water rinse in the morning to acclimatise the hands to cooler conditions. Dry well and then rub in a moisturising cream.

Composition
- 1 small cucumber.
- ½ tablespoon (8 ml) honey.
- Warm water mild soap.
- 1 tablespoon (15 ml) cornmeal.

Almonds, Manjista, and Honey Soothing Ointment

Here is a recipe from the middle ages for painfully cracked hands. Almonds are known for their mildness and softening effect on the skin. Manjista purifies blood.

- 1 ounce (30 g) ground almonds.
- 1 egg, beaten.
- ¼ ounce (7 g) ground Maddar root.
- 1 tablespoon (15 ml) honey.

Preparation

Combine well the almonds, egg, maddar root, and honey, stirring with your hands or a wooden spoon. Refrigerate.

Application

Before bed, smoothen this mixture over your hands and fingers and pull on either a pair of cotton gloves or old leather gloves. Follow this regimen for seven nights.

Shining Skin

There are two methods to make skin look beautiful and shining:

Internal Method

One should such eatable which gives tustre to the skin eg. Lemon, Carrot, Tomato, Milk etc.

External Method

One should use skin creams, oils eg. Almond oil, Olive oil, Glycerine etc.

> It has been proved that Vitamin A, C, E gives lustre and smoothness to the skin.

Seven Basic Steps to Healthy Hands

1. Eat right. Choose foods as close to the way they were "born" as possible. Vary the types of fruits and vegetables.
2. Drink at least 6 glasses of pure water a day to keep the skin moisturised inside and out.
3. Get the sleep your body needs.
4. Wear sunscreen or protective clothing to avoid overexposing. Some sunshine is necessary for the body and soul. However, today's suntan is tomorrow's ageing skin.
5. Wash with mild cleansers. Avoid extreme temperature and harsh detergents. As a normal skin function, sweat and sebaceous glands routinely rid the body of toxins and wastes.

6. Protect your hands with moisturising creams, sunscreen, or the appropriate gloves when you are exposing your hands to abrasive or outside elements.
7. Exercise. When you are faced with repetitive tasks, take time out to stretch and wiggle your fingers, wrists, hands, and arms to maintain normal range of movement.

●●

8. Feet Care

Feet carry us around and keep us mobile. Just imagine, how would we feel if we had to sit in one place all day long. So caring for the feet is very important.

Relaxing Foot Massage Oil

After washing and exercising your feet, use this fabulous aromatherapy herbal oil to further enhance your relaxed mood and soften any rough skin as well.

Composition

- 2 teaspoons (10 ml) soybean, jojoba, extra-virgin olive, or almond oil.
- 2-6 drops of (depending on desired strength) lavender, German chamomile, orange, or clay sage essential oil.

Yield

1 treatment.

Preparation

Mix all ingredients thoroughly in a small bowl.

Application

Massage onto your feet using a firm, strong hand. Apply pressure as needed to alleviate fatigue and tension in your feet. Put on socks afterwards.

Use of Flower Powder

Composition

- ¼ cup (60 ml) fine white cosmetic clay.
- ¼ cup (60 ml) cornstarch.
- 2 tablespoons (30 ml) finely ground and sifted dried lavender flowers.
- 2 tablespoons (30 ml) finely ground and sifted dried rose petals.

- 10 drops orange essential oil.
- 10 drops lavender essential oil.
- 10 drops rose or geranium essential oil.

Yield

Approximately ¾ cup (180 ml).

Preparation

Combine all ingredients in a medium-sized bowl.

Application

Sprinkle liberally on feet and legs after pedicure, sprinkle daily in your shoes, or use as a body powder.

Optional

Men can create a more masculine fragrance by omitting the floral herbs and oils and substituting 1 teaspoon (5 ml) cinnamon powder, 1 teaspoon powdered cloves, 1 teaspoon powdered all spice or nutmeg, and 30 drops orange, lemon, or lime essential oil.

Storage

Store in a shaker container or a small box with a puff in a cool, dry place.

Lavender Velvet Cream

Composition

- ½ cup (120 ml) all-vegetable shortening.
- 1 teaspoon (5 ml) beeswax.
- 3 tablespoons (45 ml) distilled water, rosewater, German chamomile tea, or lavender tea.
- 1 teaspoon (5 ml) borax.
- 15 drops lavender essential oil.
- 15 drops rose or geranium essential oil.
- 15 drops spearmint essential oil (optional, but adds a nice, mild mint note).

Yield

- Approximately ¾ cup (180 ml).

Preparation

1. In a small saucepan, heat the shortening and beeswax over low heat until just melted. Remove saucepan from heat.

2. In another small saucepan, warm the distilled water, rosewater, or tea and dissolve the borax in it; then remove saucepan from heat. (To make a herb tea to use as liquid, simply pour 1 cup [230 ml] boiling water over 1 teaspoon [5 ml] of dried herb, steep 5 to 10 minutes, then strain.
3. When both mixtures have cooled to approximately the same temperature, set the wax/shortening pan into a bowl of ice cubes and add the essential oils.
4. Drizzle the liquid into it, stirring rapidly with a small whisk or spoon. The cream should set up fairly quickly and looks and feels like fluffy cake icing.

Application

Slather it thickly onto clean feet, put on socks, and go to bed. Awaken to "feet of velvet". This product can be used wherever you have dry skin: hands, elbows, knees, or even as a cuticle conditioner. It sinks in amazingly fast, is non-greasy if you don't use too much, and makes your skin super soft.

Storage

Store in an attractive container away from heat or light. No need to refrigerate unless weather is hot. Will last approximately one year if you do choose to chill it or up to three to four months at room temperature.

Peppermint Salt Massage

Composition
- 1 tablespoon (15 ml) sea salt.
- 1 tablespoon (15 ml) extra-virgin olive oil.
- 5 drops peppermint essential oil.

Yield

1 treatment.

Preparation

In a small bowl, combine all ingredients, stirring thoroughly.

Application

Massage onto lower legs, ankles, and foot. It feels quite invigorating and refreshing and is great to use on a hot summer day!

Blister Resister Cream

Preparation

Beat ingredients together with a spoon or small whisk.

Application

Apply to blister-prone areas, and then cover with thick socks. Helps reduce friction between the sensitive spot and your shoe.

Storage

Store in a small glass or plastic jar and label. Keep it refrigerated if not to be used within thirty days.

Composition
- $1/_3$ cup (80 ml) all-vegetable shortening.
- 10 drops eucalyptus essential oil.
- 10 drops camphor essential oil.

Optional

If you're a peppermint lover, you can substitute 15 to 20 drops of peppermint essential oil instead of the above oils.

Yield

About $1/_3$ cup (80 ml).

Vanilla Foot Butter

Composition
- 4 tablespoons (60 ml) almond, olive, jojoba, soybean, or calendula oil.
- 1 vanilla bean, chopped into ¼ inch (.6 cm) pieces (available in grocery or health food stores).
- 1 tablespoon (15 ml) beeswax.
- 2 tablespoons (30 ml) cocoa butter.
- 1 tablespoon (15 ml) anhydrous lanolin.
- 20 drops geranium, rosemary, or peppermint essential oil.

Yield

Approximately ½ cup (120 ml).

Preparation
1. In a small saucepan warm the oil over low heat.
2. Add the chopped vanilla bean, cover, and allow steeping for 1 hour.
3. Remove from heat and strain. It's all right if you see tiny vanilla bean seeds—they're harmless. Save the vanilla bean for other uses.
4. Add the oil back to the pan and add the beeswax, cocoa butter, and lanolin and heat until just melted.
5. Remove from the heat and stir in essential oil if you desire. If left plain, it will smell like white chocolate, sweet and yummy!

Application
Scoop out approximately 1 teaspoon (5 ml), rub between your palms to warm and improve its spreading ability, then massage into feet as necessary to keep them wonderfully moisturised and smooth.

Storage
Store in a 4-ounce (112 g) jar. No refrigeration is necessary. This butter may harden in cold weather, but will soften upon skin contact.

Super Rich, All-Purpose Foot Cream

Here's a recipe for the thickest cream. It's got real staying power and will keep your feet the softest they've ever been. It also doubles as a fantastic lip balm and dynamite cuticle conditioner.

Composition
- 3 tablespoons (45 ml) plus 1 teaspoon (5 ml) castor oil.
- 2 teaspoons (10 ml) beeswax.
- 15 drops peppermint essential oil.
- 15 drops of rosemary essential oil.

Yield
Approximately ¼ cup (60 ml).

Preparation
1. Over very low heat, blend the castor oil and beeswax in a small saucepan, and heat until the wax is just melted. Remove from burner and allow cooling a bit.

2. Add the essential oil drops to the bottom of a 2-ounce (55 g) jar, and then pour in the oil/wax mixture.

Application

Apply enough of this wonderfully thick cream to your feet each night so that your ankles are covered as well. Put on socks.

Mineral Rich Oatmeal Soak

If you do this procedure every other day or so, you will eventually and safely remove most of the hard skin from your feet and can then reduce the treatment to twice per week. This foot-bath feels particularly good because of the oatmeal's moisturising and softening properties.

Composition
- 1 foot-bath tub.
- ½ cup (120 ml) very finely ground oatmeal.
- ¼ cup (60 ml) white cosmetic clay.
- 5 drops geranium, lavender, or eucalyptus essential oil (optional), pumice stone or foot file.

Yield

1 treatment.

Preparation

1. To make the ground oatmeal, put about ¾ cup (180 ml) old-fashioned "grocery store" variety oatmeal into a food processor and process until the oats are of a powder-like consistency.
2. Place a towel on the floor in front of the chair where you will be sitting as you soak your feet. Pour enough water into the tub (whatever temperature you desire) so that your ankles will be covered. Slowly stir in the oatmeal and clay until dissolved, then add essential oil if you desire.

Application

1. Soak your feet for at least 10 to 15 minutes or until your calluses are soft, but not until your feet are "puny".
2. Very gently scrub your calluses and/or corns with the pumice stone or file just until the top layer of tough dead skin has been removed.

3. Rinse, and then roughly dry with a coarse towel.
4. Apply a heavy cream.

Caution: Diabetics should not soak their feet. Most of them suffer from circulatory disorders and cannot feel if the water temperature is too hot or cold. Additionally, if the foot skin gets too soft as a result of soaking, it can lead to pre-ulcerations especially between the toes in the web spaces.

Benefits of Barefoot Walking

The best treatment for feet encased in shoes all day is to go barefoot. One-fifth of the world's population never wears shoes—ever! But when people who usually go barefoot begin to wear shoes, their feet begin to suffer. As often as possible, walk barefoot on the beach, in your yard, or at least around the house. Walking on the grass or sand massages your feet, strengthens your muscles and feels very relaxing.

Care of Tired Feet

- ◆ Walking bare foot on grass early in the morning when grass is wet with night dew is said to be useful for feet and is very relaxing.
- ◆ Put your feet in warm water containing Salt and Lemon. This will give relaxing mode to your feet and shine to skin.

Caution

Please be very careful if you're diabetic. Walk only on clean surface to avoid cutting and puncturing your feet.

If you can cut short on wearing shoes by 30 percent, you will save wear and tear on your feet and extend the life of your shoes!

●●

9. Hair Care

The face of an individual is a personal identity in which hair plays a significant role. Therefore, a perfect head with hair is an attribute of personality and beauty. Ayurveda states the following qualities of good hair:

Healthy Hair (Prashastha Kesha)
Every strand of hair should be long, black, soft, shiny and strong. Genetically Indians are black haired and a dark head is any time better and goes well on any dress.

In order to know how to keep one's hair healthy and wealthy, one should have knowledge about the factors responsible for hair growth, fall, and other hair problems. In brief, it can be stated that hair reflects the inside story of a person, as well as his/her general state of health. Because of growing importance of hair care, a new branch of cosmetology called 'TRICHOLOGY' has come up, especially dealing in the science and study of hair or more specifically the science of the physical, emotional and environmental causes of hair and scalp maladies. The name comes from the Greek word 'trichos', which means hair.

Factors Responsible for Hair Problems
- Age.
- General state of health.
- Environment.
- Lifestyle.
- Nutrition and exercise.

Hair Composition
Hair contains ninety seven percent protein and three percent moisture. This strong fibrous protein called keratin also comprises our nails. These two agents are most useful in treating hair structure, both internally and externally.

Protein-> to strengthen and fortify.
Moisture-> to hydrate.

Each hair is an incredibly strong and resistant fibre, having a complete structure, which can be altered by our daily activities like washing, drying, blow-drying, and chemically changing colour and texture.

Characteristics of Good Hair
1. Quite elastic, can stretch up to 30 percent beyond its normal length and spring back.
2. The ability to absorb and hold moisture up to 50% of its weight, called 'porosity'.

Test Your Own Hair
1. Carefully stretch a strand between your thumb and index finger.
2. Release the tension on the strand and see if the hair returns to its normal length.
3. If it does not or if it breaks, the hair has poor elasticity.
4. This indicates that your hair is brittle and lacks moisture.

The Sink or Float Test
To test porosity of the hair.
- Pick up one hair each from the top, back and two sides of your head.
- Drop these strands into a bowel of water.
- If they sink within 5 to 10 seconds your hair is overly porous.
- Such hair is very fragile and should be conditioned thoroughly.

Hair Analysis
Many toxins as well as drugs that we ingest show up in our hair. Hair analysis can uncover some conditions that conventional medical testing cannot.

The Root of the Matter
Each hair comes out of the scalp through the hair follicle. The angle at which the hair comes out of the skin is directly related to the

shape of the hair. **Straight hair** is round in cross section and shoots straight out from the scalp. **Wavy hair** is oval in shape and comes out of the scalp at a slight angle. **Curly hair** is flattened and comes out of the scalp at an extreme angle.

Each hair has its own blood, nerve, and muscle supply, found within the dermal layer of the skin. At the base of the hair follicle, embedded in the dermis, is the papilla, the "root" through which a rich supply of oxygenated blood feeds hair growth via blood capillaries. Blood is the communication link between the body and the hair. Imbalances or toxicity in the body are interpreted and transferred to the hair through the blood supply—or not transferred, as the case may be, such as in a sluggish or blocked flow of blood. Stress, pollutants taken into the body, hormonal fluctuations, illnesses, pharmaceutical or illicit drugs, and poor diet all come into play in this integral part of nourishing hair growth. The hair bulb envelops the hair papilla. If a hair is pulled out from the root, it is the hair bulb that you see at the end of the strand. Just as a beautiful flower sprouts forth and grows from a bulb within rich fertile soil, so does the hair germinate in and sprout from the hair bulb, growing prolifically with the papilla's rich source of nutrients.

Don't Sweat It!

Hair too faces problems—the wind messes it up, the atmosphere does its share, and so do our glands. Glands are found in the dermal layer of the skin. Glands are of two types—sweat glands, which secrete a watery fluid (perspiration), and sebaceous glands, which secrete a fatty substance called sebum.

The Sweat Glands

Secretions from the sweat glands are one of the three ways by which we eliminate toxins from our body (the other two are bowel movement and urination). The body has about two million sweat glands, and they come in two types: the eccrine and the apocrine glands.

1. Eccrine sweat glands

In the simplest of terms, the eccrine glands are responsible for secreting the sweat that bathes our skin in moisture, maintains an acid-balanced environment that prevents the proliferation of undesirable bacteria or fungi. We normally excrete 1 to 2.6 pints (800 to 1,230 ml) of water during 24 hours—but this amount can increase tenfold when we perspire heavily. Perspiration from the eccrine glands also regulates our body temperature by evaporating from the skin, cooling us off when we're overheated. Stress and pungent, spicy foods will also increase the eccrine glands' flow of sweat. Sweat is comprised of water, sodium salts, potassium, sulphuric acid, iron, phosphorus, lactic acid, and urea (a toxic by-product of animal protein metabolism that is processed by the kidneys). The skin will also secrete ingested poisons (heavy metals, arsenic, and so on) if the body's vital functions are all healthy.

2. Apocrine sweat glands

Body odour is secreted from our apocrine glands, and they are scattered around our body, in our armpits, on our face, chest, and pubic and anal areas. These glands empty into the hair follicles near the skin surface. Our personal scents change according to our state of health and mind. For example, meat eaters have a dramatically different smell. Stress can greatly alter the nature of our body aroma as well as increase the amount of secretion, because the adrenal glands, when stressed, will increase the output of the male sex hormone androgen (which is responsible for controlling the apocrine glands). The odour is accentuated further by the secretions from the sebaceous glands—sebum—which is a fatty, oily substance that the odours from the apocrine glands cling to when deposited on the scalp and hair. Sebum will absorb odours such as smoke and perfume, as well as any of the more pleasant essential oil fragrances that you may massage into your hair and scalp.

The Sebaceous Glands

The sebaceous glands are the body's built-in automatic lubrication system. There are about 100 such glands per sq. inch of skin, heavily concentrated on the scalp, face, and upper torso. Pituitary, thyroid, and sex gland hormones primarily regulate them. They secrete sebum, which serves as a protective mantle for the outer skin and hair and keeps the hair shiny and moist. In puberty the sebaceous glands tend to work overtime, causing skin and hair problems; hair and skin care formulas with astringent qualities will modify and balance such an overabundance of sebum. Conversely, a smooth, consistent secretion of sebum and sweat may be altered and blocked by certain hormonal conditions, age, inadequate diet, and stress. Whether you're experiencing too much or too little sebum, an assessment of your lifestyle and activities, including diet, exercise, and stress, is in order. It is very important to stay the course with gentle, natural, and preferably organic products for the hair and skin.

Hair Growth

Hair is amazing in its prolific growth. In fact, its rate of cell production in the body is second only to that of bone marrow! Our hair grows approximately ½ inch (13 mm) a month, and sometimes slightly faster. When we're highly active, growth usually slows, and we may even begin to experience hair loss. The active growing phase of an individual hair is called anlagen phase, and it could grow 18 to 30 inches (45 to 75 cm) through this period. The hair then goes into an intermediate or transitional phase called the cartage phase just before entering the tillage phase, in which it rests for about a hundred days, and then falls out. About 85 to 90 percent of all the hair on the head is in an active growing phase at any given moment, while 10 to 15 percent is resting. Each hair grows at different rates. Under normal healthy conditions, you don't need to be concerned that they will rest and fall out at the same time.

Aloe vera material obtain after scraping the skin when dissolved in ethyl alcohol (alcohol), used as hair dye to stimulate hair growth.

Alopecia or Hair Loss

Hair loss, also known as *alopecia*, is quite common. You can lose approximately 50 to 100 hairs a day and feel fairly confident that it is normal. However, if you experience a steady loss of more than this, it is important to see a trichologist or a medical doctor to have the situation diagnosed. Sudden onset of hair loss can be discussed with a professional. Hair loss may be temporary depending on its cause, such as if it were caused by illness or a dramatic change in diet, or taking or stopping a given medication. The body eventually balances itself, and hair growth should return to normal.

Diffusion of hair loss, which may occur all over the head or in patches, is not possible to correct or balance itself without qualified help. It will not be cured until its cause—often found to include a hormonal imbalance or mineral deficiency, or anemia—is diagnosed and treated.

Permanent hair loss can result from genetic factors, such as male or female pattern of baldness, as well as specific forms of alopecia, especially traction alopecia.

Possible causes of hair loss
- Hormonal imbalances.
- Anaemia.
- Mineral imbalances.
- Exposure to poisons (heavy metals, pesticides, and so on).
- X-rays.
- Many forms of drugs.
- Liver and kidney disease.
- Autoimmune disease.
- Stress.
- Poor diet, including severe forms of food deprivation such as anorexia nervosa.
- Genetic, hereditary thinning or balding (androgenetic alopecia).

Possible causes of hair breakage
- Inherited hair defects (rare).
- Fungal infections, such as ringworm.
- Chemical or mechanical damage or both (from permanent relaxes or waves, or colour treatments).
- Excessive exposure to sunlight.
- Poor diet.

Possible causes of bald patches
- Alopecia (sudden hair loss in round patches), which may be triggered by many factors, including stress, viral or bacterial infection, anaemia, and trauma.
- Trichotillomania (the pulling out of your own hair).
- Ringworm (a fungal infection).
- Genetic baldness.
- Hairstyles worn very tightly over long periods of time, such as braids or ponytails (also known as traction alopecia).

Choosing the Right Herbal Cosmetics for Hair Care

Hair care products are a multibillion-dollar worldwide industry; whether you're strolling through the local drugstore, supermarket, health food store, or your favourite salon, the selection of hair care formulas can be quite confusing, to say the least. There are so many of them! How do you choose the ones that will be the best for your hair?

Qualities of an Ideal Hair Product

According to this list of desirable attributes, we want products that:
- Cleanse without stripping natural oils.
- Replace lost protein, moisture, and nutrients.
- Increase and fortify the strength and elasticity of the hair.
- Protect the hair cuticle.
- Condition without "weighing down" the hair or building up on the scalp.
- Even out porosity and prevent moisture loss.
- Smooth abraded cuticle scales and lock in moisture while creating brilliant shine.
- Prevent intense drying from the environment through the use of sunscreens.
- Give an exceptional tactile quality or "feel" to the hair.

Common Herbs Used in Hair Care

	Common name	Latin name
1.	Kikar	Acacia arabica
2.	Shikakai	Acacia concinna
3.	Burdock	Arcticum lappa
4.	Arnica	Arnica montana
5.	Birch	Betula pendula
6.	Marigold	Calendula officinalis
7.	Safflower	Carthamus tinctoria
8.	Brahmi	Centella aciatica
9.	Nariyal	Cocos nucifera
10.	Bihi	Cydinia oblonga

11.	Bhangra	Eclipta alba
12.	Patang	Haematoxylon camp
13.	Akhrot	Jiptuglans regia
14.	Mehndi	Lawsonia inermis
15.	Shahtoot	Morus Alba
16.	Jatamansi	Nardostachys jatamansi
17.	Amla	Phyllanthus emblica
18.	Jaborandi	Pilocarpus jaborandi
19.	Narra	Pterrocarpus indica
20.	Bacho	Rubia tinctorum
21.	Ritha	Sapindus mukorrossi
22.	Kust	Saussurea lappa
23.	Til	Sesamum indicum
24.	Behera	Terminalia belerica
25.	Banajwain	Thymus serphyllum
26.	Giloe	Tinospora cordifolia
27.	Methi	Trigonella foenum graecum
28.	Stinging nettle	Utrica dioica

Assessing Your Hair Condition

Hair can be oily and dry at the same time, and so can the scalp. The hair and scalp are in fact always changing—according to the seasons, according to hormonal fluctuations, according to changes in lifestyle or nutrition, and so on. If your hair is colour treated, you could have dry, damaged ends and an oily scalp. In a case like this—as in any instance where there are dramatic differences between hair and scalp conditions—you'll need to strike a balance, treating the oily scalp without accentuating the dry hair condition.

Normal Hair

We all would like to say our hair is normal. The word 'normal', however, is a specific term used to describe hair that is strong, resilient, moisturised, and shiny—whether fine, medium, or coarse in diameter, and straight, wavy, or curly in its shape or textural movement. A normal scalp is one that is moist and pink without having any form of irritation, redness or bumps (these may be symptoms of folliculate, an irritation of the hair follicles). The goal of normal hair and scalp is to maintain this balanced state.

Oily Hair

Oily hair is not very prevalent today because of the amount of shampooing that we do, which keeps excess sebum at bay. Oily hair usually means oily scalp. Fine hair tends to take on a limp, greasy look if the sebaceous glands are working overtime. Adolescents often experience this condition; however, the hormones do balance and normalise over time, given a healthy diet and lifestyle. In all cases of oily scalp it is important to choose a gentle cleansing shampoo that will wash away excess oil without exacerbating the problem. It is quite possible that you will need to select a shampoo for any oily scalp while choosing a conditioner for dry hair.

Dry Hair

Dry hair is dull, lacklustre, and, at the extreme, brittle in its appearance. This type of hair feels hard, not soft and silky. It craves moisture, and in most instances requires a healthy dose of protein. Dry hair needs protection in the form of emollients and lubricants, which will lay down the outside cuticle layer of the hair and create shine. Humectants will attract and retain moisture within this type of hair.

Hair may be dry for a variety of reasons. This may be a natural condition of the hair, especially with very curly or frizzy hair. Dryness can also be created by the products used on the hair—shampoos, styling products, and the like. It can occur after mechanical treatment of the hair, such as styling or chemically treating with colour, waves, or relaxes, or as a response to environmental conditions like sun, chlorine, salt water, or forced heat in cold climates. A dry scalp can be created by harsh products used on the hair, or by not thoroughly rinsing products out of the hair and off the scalp. Many people who think they have dandruff don't have dandruff at all—they simply have flaking scalp from a buildup of dry cells, mixed with shampoo and conditioner residue that has not been thoroughly rinsed from the hair. A thorough massaging of the scalp by shampoo is absolutely necessary to remove this buildup.

Hormonal and environmental conditions can certainly create as well as aggravate a dry scalp. And a dry scalp can be an internally created condition, if your diet does not include enough of the essential fatty acids and vitamins to maintain a moisturised, lubricated skin. Shampoos and conditioners chosen for dry hair and scalp conditions need to be quite nutritive in nature to smoothen the hair and build its strength, while adding moisture.

Combinations

Following are some of the more common hair and scalp combinations which guide you to assess your own hair and scalp types and then select wisely from the hair care products available. Remember that normal, oily, or dry conditions may occur on fine, medium, and coarse hair types. It's all relative.

1. **Normal scalp and hair:** It is desirable to maintain this balanced healthy state with a regular daily cleansing and conditioning routine.
2. **Oily scalp and hair:** Try not to overstimulate the scalp with aggressive manipulation or products, so as not to create extra sebum production. Gently cleanse every day. Try to minimise the amount of styling products you use.
3. **Oily scalp and dry hair:** Gently cleanse every day with a cleanser for normal to oily hair types. Another option you'll find is a balancing shampoo for normal hair. Alternate this at least once a week with a purifying shampoo. Apply a moisturising conditioner of any type specifically to your hair areas.
4. **Dry scalp and hair:** Daily cleansing and conditioning with moisturising and emollient treatments will go a long way towards alleviating a dry, tight scalp, while replenishing lost moisture and proteins along the hair shaft.
5. **Oily scalp and normal hair:** Treat the oily scalp condition as outlined above while using a conditioner throughout the lengths of hair.
6. **Dry scalp and normal hair:** Use rich, nourishing shampoos that are moisturising on the scalp. Generally these will be designated as shampoos for dry hair or for normal to dry hair types.

Quick Tips for Shampooing

- When shampooing and rinsing, always work from the scalp area out to the ends. This is the direction of the cuticle scales.
- Try not to cluster or bunch longer lengths of hair as you massage; this can cause tangling.
- Don't vigorously rub the hair against itself while you shampoo or condition. This will roughen and stress the hair shaft, particularly the cuticle scales.

Hair Cosmetic Recipes

Here are some Herbal Cosmetic Recipes for healthy hair.

Pure shampoo

The ingredients for this recipe are chosen for their desirable aromatic flavour.

Composition
- 1-2 tablespoons (15-30 ml) dried herbs of your choice. Select any one or two from the list on pages 79 and 80.
- 8 ounces (235 ml) purified water.
- 2 ounces (60 ml) liquid glycerin soap.
- 1 teaspoon (5 ml) base oil of your choice (eliminate or reduce for oily conditions; increase for dry).
- 15-60 drops essential oils of your choice, as conditions require.

Yield

8-10 ounces (235-295 ml).

Preparation

1. Prepare a decoction or infusion of your desired herb or combinations of herbs. Remember that a decoction is used for roots, stems, and seeds, or more fibrous, tough plants, while infusions are used for more delicate plant parts, including leaves and flowers. If you are combining herbs that need different treatments, decoct and infuse them separately, then mix these liquids.

   For a decoction, place the herbs in water in a stainless steel or glass pan. Bring to boil, reduce the heat, and simmer on lowflame for up to 10 minutes. Remove from the heat, let the mixture cool, strain off the liquid, and discard the spent herbs.

For an infusion, bring the water to boil. Place the herbs in a stainless steel or glass pan and pour the boiling water over them. Let steep for at least 20 minutes, then let the mixture cool (if it isn't cool already), strain off the liquid, and discard the spent herbs.

Tip

To increase the potency of the formula, let the herbs steep in the cooled liquid in an airtight container for a couple of days before straining and using.

2. Mix the herbal infusion or decoction with the soap, base oil, and desired essential oils. Shake well. Refrigerate the shampoo between uses, for up to a week.

Application

Use the formula for every shampoo. Shake well before each use.

You can also add ingredients with properties suitable for your particular hair condition, such as apple juice, honey, egg, aloe-vera, gelatin, and glycerin or lecithin. *(See pages 115 to 121.)*

Use 1 tablespoon (15 ml) per shampoo formula.

Pure Shampoo for Different Conditions

This gives you a framework to make your own formulae. It is not necessary for you to use the ingredients outlined. If you choose to decoct only one specific herb for a given condition and add one flavoured essential oil, that's perfectly all right. The fact that you are using a pure shampoo with no chemicals in it is the first step toward becoming as creative as you would like. Also remember that you can do something as simple as purchasing a pure shampoo and add healthy ingredients as required—such as essential oils, egg, or gelatin. *Remember to complete a patch test before using your hair care formula.*

To kill Hair Lice

Hair lice is a common problem and synthetic method are available to combat it. But it can be controlled by using plant *"Annona Squamosa* (Sharifa). Paste of seed or leaf applied on hair for killing lice. Wash it down after an hour.

Condition	Herbs to decoct or infuse	Base oils	Essential oils
Normal hair	Rosemary, amla	Almond oil plus up to 1 tablespoon (15 ml) of aloe-vera	Bergamot, orange, rose
Dry hair	Lavender, bhringraj	Jojoba oil plus up to 1 tablespoon (15 ml) of aloe-vera and lecithin (drizzle into warmed formula)	Carrot seed, clary sage, geranium, jasmine
Oily hair	Lemon grass, thyme	Almond oil	Basil (tulsi), peppermint, rosemary
Sensitive scalp (dandruff, dermatitis, inflammation)	Triphala (amla+ harda+ bibitaki)	Jojoba or castor oil	Rosemary, sage, tea tree
Hair loss or thinning	Basil, rosemary, sage	Jojoba oil	Basil, lemon

Herbal/Natural Shampoos

- **Regular shampoo:** Use of home-made mixture of shikakai, reetha, and amla in equal ratio gives hair better appearance than shampoos and it is also devoid of ill effects on the hair.
- **Protein shampoo:** Apply the white part of egg once a week to your hair; it provides protein to the hair root.
- **Health shampoo:** Take reetha, shikakai, multani mitti, nagarmotha, mehndi, and amla in equal quantities. Soak it in water overnight and make a paste out of it the next morning. Use this paste to wash your hair. This is one of the best shampoos.
- **Hair fall preventive shampoo:** Paste of flower of til (sesame) and gokharu in cow milk should be applied for seven continuous days. This stops hair loss and encourages growth.

- **Colour-improving paste:** Soak mehndi in water overnight, and boil it until it becomes paste. Apply it on the hair and wait until it dries up before washing it with water only. Do this process once in a week. This improves hair colour and shine.
- **Natural shampoos:** Nature has an abundance of goodness stored in products like shikakai and reetha. They act as cleansing agents, while henna is a good conditioner. Soaps don't clean your hair effectively since they leave behind fine granule deposits of calcium and magnesium, leading to an unhealthy scalp. Soaps strip your hair of natural oils, making hair look dry and lifeless. The pH level of your hair is neutral while soaps have a pH level of about 10, making them highly alkaline. Hair requires as much high quality care as skin does to keep it healthy.

Hair Rinses

Herbal hair rinses are natural conditioners and serve a variety of functions. When applied through your hair after shampooing they will close down the cuticle, creating exceptionally smooth and shiny hair that feels thicker and is more manageable. Hair rinses can also be quite therapeutic for the scalp. They can bring to hair an acid-balanced pH, remove soap residue, and enhance colour.

A hair rinse may be as simple as adding a few drops of an essential oil to your final rinse of water for its aromatic and therapeutic value, or as complex as creating a medicinal rinse that combines several herbs and essential oils. Many options exist. The type of rinse that you choose to make will depend on how creative you want to get. It depends on your condition or problem. Again, you may refer to the list of essential oils, and natural ingredients that resonate with your needs and desires.

When Should One Rinse?

- If you have normal to dry hair, use the rinse before applying a conditioner.
- If you have oily hair, use the rinse after applying a conditioner.

Rinse Recipes

Shikakai hair wash

Powder equal quantities of the following ingredients, mix them together and bottle them up. Use it alongwith the requisite amount of water for cleaning and washing hair.

Composition

1. Shikakai pods.
2. Green grams.
3. Dried amla.
4. Dried curry leaves.
5. Dried lime peel.
6. Fenugreek seeds
   (Methi leaves).

Dandruff hair wash

Make fine powder of (in equal quantity):
1. Shikakai.
2. Reetha.
3. Rind of lemon and orange.
4. Layer of Nimba tree bark (Margosa).
5. Mehndi.
6. Chandan.
7. Daru haridra.
8. Saindhava lavana.

Application

5 to 6 tsp of this powder in 2 cups of water is soaked at night. In the morning, boil this mixture till it forms a paste. Wet hair and apply all over scalp. After 10 to 15 minutes, cleanse the scalp thoroughly.

Shikakai application as natural hair wash is always after an oil massage of scalp. Only then do the saponins and the active ingredients in the material go into the layers of the skin, soften the tissues and activate the cells. If the bath is taken without using oil we will be getting only part of its action.

Do's
- Wash hair regularly, with herbal solution prepared by boiling Neem leaves in water.
- Washing hair twice a day is effective in the condition. After washing, the hair should be completely dried. Massage scalp with warm oil at night.

Don'ts

Avoid over-application of oil on scalp; avoid soap and shampoo that are chemically prepared.

Herbal Infusion Rinse

You can use these suggested herbs singly or in combination.

a. Herbs for normal hair

Chamomile, rosemary, sage, bhringraj, amla.

b. Herbs for oily hair

Lemongrass, mint, and thyme.

c. Herbs for dry hair

Lavender, jasmine, orange, rose, sandalwood, carrot seed.

Composition
- 2 tablespoons (30 ml) dried herbs (as suggested above).
- 1 cup (250 ml) purified water.
- 3-5 drops essential oils of your choice (optional).

Yield

1 treatment

Preparation

1. Bring the water to a boil. Place the herbs in a stainless steel or glass pan and pour the boiling water over them. Let it steep for 10-15 minutes.
2. Drain off the liquid and discard the spent herbs. Mix in the essential oil and then use immediately.

Tea Tree Rinse

The following herbal combination is antiseptic, astringent, and soothing. Tea tree essential oil is antifungal and antiseptic and so very effective for scalp problems that have a fungal or bacterial origin. It is used for sensitive itchy scalp.

Composition
- 2 cups (500 ml) purified or distilled water.
- 1 heaped tablespoon (15 ml, or about 1 handful) each of dried triphala, haridra, nimba, khadir and rind of lemon or orange decoction.
- 1 drop tea tree essential oil (optional).
- 1 drop lavender essential oil.

Yield
1-3 treatments, depending on hair length.

Preparation
Place the herbs in the water in a stainless steel or glass pan. Bring to a boil, then immediately remove from the heat. Let the "tea" sit overnight, then strain out the herbs.

Application
After shampooing with a gentle shampoo and rinsing thoroughly, apply the herbal tea as your final rinse.

Lemon Juice Highlighting Rinse
The rinse makes the hair very shiny, and is great for bringing out highlights in light brown hair—although it's wonderful for all hair colours. It is most beneficial for normal to oily hair conditions.

Composition
- 2 lemons.
- 2 cups (500 ml) purified water.

Yield
1 treatment.

Preparation and Application
Squeeze the juice from the lemons into the water. The formula accentuates the acidification of both hair and scalp, softening and subtly lightening the hair.

Purifying and Stimulating Hair and Scalp Rinse
This herbal vinegar rinse has a soothing and detoxifying effect on

the hair and scalp while it increases blood circulation to the hair follicles.

Composition
- 2 tablespoons (30 ml) dried mint.
- 2 tablespoons (30 ml) dried basil.
- 2 tablespoons (30 ml) dried rosemary.
- 2 tablespoons (30 ml) dried sage.
- 3-5 drops essential oils of your choice (try a few drops each of lavender and peppermint).
- 2 cups (500 ml) organic apple cider vinegar.

Yield
Approximately 15 treatments.

Preparation
1. Chop the herbs. Place them in a wide mouthed quart (1 litre) glass jar and pour in the apple cider vinegar, making sure that the herbs are completely covered (add more vinegar if necessary). Gently stir, and then cover. If you're using a metal lid, place plastic wrap or wax paper over the opening first, then cover so that the vinegar doesn't corrode the metal.
2. Let the herbs steep in the vinegar for up to two weeks at room temperature. Then strain off the liquid, discard the spent herbs, and store the vinegar in a dark glass bottle in a cool, dark place. This remedy can be kept for up to a year.

Application
Add 2 tablespoons (30 ml) of the herbal vinegar to 1 cup (250 ml) of warm water and massage it onto the scalp after shampooing. Do not rinse out. Repeat once every week.

Hair Colour Rinses

Use the following herbal decoctions as colour-enhancing rinses after shampooing and rinsing. Towel-dry hair, then flow the rinse through it. Do not rinse out.
- For enhancing bold hair, decoct calendula and chamomile.
- For enhancing dark hair, decoct rosemary, sage, or black tea.
- For enhancing red hair, decoct sandalwood (for reddish brown tones) or saffron (for copper tones).

Hair And Scalp Conditioners

Conditioning treatments strengthen and moisturise the hair, complementing the acidifying nature of hair rinses. Depending on the treatment, they can be applied before or after shampooing and can be rinsed out or left in. Generally, the longer conditioners are left in, the more powerful are their effects.

Multi-Purpose Conditioner

This conditioner is especially good for maintaining healthy, normal hair in its optimal condition. Aloe-vera has tremendous moisturising properties, while lemon juice is quite purifying and cleaning. Take lavender, rosemary, or mint essential oils, depending upon whether you're seeking a relaxing or stimulating effect.

Composition
- ¼ cup (60 ml) aloe-vera gel.
- ½ lemon.
- 3-5 drops essential oils of your choice.

Yield

1 treatment.

Preparation

Mix the aloe-vera gel with the juice of half a lemon. Add the essential oils.

Application

Apply to freshly shampooed hair. Leave on for 3 to 5 minutes, then rinse thoroughly.

Stimulating Ginger Elixir Scalp Treatment

Ginger is considered one of the most powerful herbs in Ayurveda. It has potent stimulating properties. It increases the blood circulation. This is an excellent moisturising scalp conditioning formula, which can stimulate hair growth.

Composition
- 1 tablespoon (15 ml) finely grated ginger.
- 1 tablespoon (15 ml) sesame or jojoba oil.

Yield
   1 treatment.

Preparation and Application
   This formula can be applied after shampooing. If applied, be sure to rinse extremely well. Combine the ingredients, massage into the scalp, and leave on for at least 30 minutes. (You can leave on overnight to receive the maximum benefit.) Rinse out with tepid water.

Stimulating Conditioner for all Hair Types
Follow the same directions as above, but instead of floral herbs substitute the aromatic basil, and rosemary. Also, add essential oils of bergamot, clary sage, and geranium. These herbs and oils have a refreshing, stimulating aroma.

Moisturising Banana Hair Conditioner
High in vitamins, and minerals, bananas are very effective humectants and moisturisers. Couple this with honey and sweet almond oil and you have a match made in heaven.

Composition
- 1 small, ripe organic banana.
- 1 tablespoon (15 ml) organic honey.
- 1 teaspoon (15 ml) sweet almond oil.

Yield
   1 treatment.

Preparation and Application
   Mash the banana together with the honey and sweet almond oil. Apply this mixture to your shampooed hair. Cover your hair with a plastic bag to allow for body heat to accentuate the conditioning effect, and leave the mixture on for 15 to 30 minutes. Rinse thoroughly.

Natural, Organic Hair Colours
Currently, there's been a major resurgence of pure vegetable hair colouring products. Primary among these is henna. Whether applied in the salon or at home, many top-quality pure vegetable hair colours and hennas are now available to colour the hair.

As with chemical colour treatments, it is very important that anyone using vegetable-based dyes, also use gentle shampoos and conditioner. Protein and moisturising treatments should be applied regularly to maintain the tone and reflective shine that the colour has given and to prevent the colour from fading too quickly.

Henna: The Non-toxic Approach to Hair Colour

Since ancient times, the leaves and stems of the henna plant (Lawsonis inermis) have been used as hair cosmetics. Lawsone produces a red colour in the hair. A wide range of colours can be achieved, from blondes to reds to browns to blacks, by mixing the henna leaves and stems with other plant dye materials. Natural henna, which has no colouring properties, comes from the crushed stems of the shrub and is an excellent conditioning and modifying ingredient in shampoos and rinses. Depending on where each batch of henna comes from and when it was harvested, the strength of its properties may be subtly different.

When henna is applied to hair, it envelops and stains each hair strand, not only tinting the hair but also giving it an incredible feeling of fullness and a highly reflective shine. The results will depend on the type of henna you choose, the colour, condition, and porosity of your hair, and the amount of time that you leave it in your hair. Henna is often termed a progressive dye because each additional application increases the absorption. In other words, the more often you use henna, the more penetrating the results will be.

Henna Combinations

When mixed with other plant dye materials, henna treatments can produce a wide range of colours. To combine these plant materials with your henna, make a decoction or infusion, as noted, and substitute the hebraized liquid with the water called for in your henna formula preparation instructions. Adjust these proportions according to your desired results and the amount you need.

Plant	Part used	Preparation per ½ cup (120 ml) water	Colouring Effect
Chamomile, Roman or German	Flowers	Infusion: 2 tablespoons (30 ml)	Will accentuate honey highlights.
Rhubarb	Root	Decoction: 2 tablespoons (30 ml)	Will create golden yellow tones.
Saffron	Stigma from flower	Infusion: 2 grams	This may be a costly proposition, because saffron is very expensive, but it also serves as an excellent dye and will accentuate yellow.
Madder (Manjista)	Root	Decoction: 2 tablespoons (30 ml)	Will accentuate red tones.
Alkanet	Root	Decoction: 1 tablespoon (15 ml)	Will accentuate red brown tones.
Sandalwood	Heartwood	Decoction: 2 tablespoons (30 ml)	Will accentuate reddish brown tones.
Rosemary	Leaves	Infusion: 2 tablespoons (30 ml)	Will accentuate brown shades.
Sage	Leaves	Infusion: 2 tablespoons (30 ml)	Will accentuate brown shades.
Walnut	Leaves	Infusion: 1 tablespoon (15 ml)	Will accentuate brown shades.
Walnut	Husks	Decoction: 1 tablespoon (15 ml)	Will accentuate and enrich dark brown shades.
Indigo	Leaves	Infusion: 1 tablespoon (15 ml)	Will accentuate lustrous blue-black tonality.

Shikakai Hair Wash

Powder equal quantities of the following ingredients. Mix them together and keep in a bottle. Use it along with the requisite amount of water for cleaning and washing hair.

Composition
- Shikakai pods.
- Green grams.
- Dried amla.
- Dried curry leaves.
- Dried lime peel.
- Fenugreek seeds.

Kesh Raj Hair Oil

Herbal hair care tonic, Kesh Raj (external application) promotes hair growth, prevents hair fall and allergies.

Hair fall is a disorder and common problem these days that is predominant in all age groups and in both sexes. This may be due to several factors, viz. pollution (water, air), food adulteration, drug reaction, anxiety, mental tensions, disturbed metabolism, stress etc. All these mainly act on the hair follicles and make them lose their lustre and rejuvenating capacity. Moreover, the shampoos available in the market aggravate the situation rather than alleviate it. The herbal hair oil works on the roots of the hair, strengthens and replenishes the follicles and rejuvenates them and results in not only stoppage of hair fall but also helps in hair growth.

Composition
1. Bhringraj/Bharangaraj 1 kg.
2. Mendhi/Mehndi (Lawsonia inermis) 1 kg.
3. Amlaki/Amla (Emblica officinalis) 1 kg.
4. Vasaka/Bansa (Adhatoda vasica) 1 kg.
5. Kamboji/Kuchandan (Adenanthera pavonina) 1 kg.

All these herbs are made into a paste and mixed with 4 litres of gingelly (sesame) oil/coconut oil and heated gently until the water content in the mixture evaporates. The best oil for a base is sesame. (Do not boil this or you will burn the herbs). To the above oil, add the following powders/paste.

1. Kachura   100 gm.
2. Usheera   100 gm.
3. Chandan   100 gm.
4. Musta   100 gm.

Thoroughly mix the ingredients in the oil and heat over a gentle flame. Keep the container in an unheated oven for a day or two. Later, strain the oil and pour into a good bottle.

Popular Hair (Growth) Tonics

Many herbals are used in hair tonics and hair growth oils. The leaf juices of bhringraj can be combined with any of the following, and can be prepared as explained above.

1. Japa (flowers)
2. Jasmine (flowers)
3. Kamboji
4. Vasaka
5. Mehndi
6. Fruit of amla
7. Medhika/castor
8. Kachura
9. Ananthamula
10. Jatamamsi

They are used in the preparation of hair oils. These are processed with expressed juices, decoctions or pastes of medicinal herbs for different applications. For example:

1. The use of castor oil for cooling.
2. The use of gingelly oil for softening the tissues on the scalp.
3. The use of coconut oil for lubrication and nourishment.
4. The use of bhringraj, japa and mehndi brings out a luxuriant hair growth and slowly improves the melanin formation by the melanocytes.
5. Amla imparts a cooling effect and prevents allergic reactions and is also used as a conditioner.
6. Vasa, methika and bhringraj prevent/cure dandruff and retain the natural colour of hair.

Bhringamlaka Hair Oil

Composition

1. Fresh juice of bhringraj   500 ml.
2. Fresh juice of amlaki   500 ml.
3. Coconut oil (base)   500 ml.
4. Cow's milk   2500 ml.
5. Powder of yastimadhu   10 grams

Preparation

All the above liquids (1 to 3) are mixed well in a clean steel vessel and cow's milk (2.5 litres) should be added and heated gently until the water content in the mixture evaporates. To this oil add 10 grams of yastimadhu powder. Thoroughly mix the ingredients in the oil again and heat on gentle flame for 2 minutes and remove from stove. Keep the vessel in an unheated oven for a day. Later, strain oil and pour into a bottle and use.

Nili Bhringa Hair Oil

Composition

1. Nili leaves' fresh juice   768 ml.
2. Bhringraj fresh juice   768 ml.
3. Indra varuni fresh juice   768 ml.
4. Amlaki fresh juice   768 ml.
5. Goat's milk   768 ml.
6. Coconut milk   768 ml.
7. Cow's milk   768 ml.
8. Coconut oil (base)   768 ml.
9. Yastimadhu   32 grams
10. Gunja mula (root)   32 grams

Prepare oil as described above and use. It is a good hair darkener and tonic.

To make Hair Dark

There are so many methods to make hair dark but natural methods are rare. Henna is one of the methods to make hair dark or brown and no doubt it is good for hair conditioning.

A plant *Salvia Officinalis* (Family — Labiatae) can be used to darken the hair. In this method 15 grams of *Salvia Officinalis* is taken into one litre water. Steep leaves in water for two hours then strain. Pour over hairs and leave on for half an hour then rinse out.

Hamdard Dawakhana preparation for Hair Problems

Hamdard Preparation (Herbal)

- Jula-mula preparation contains Amla, Sikakaii, Sarson and other herbs. It brings lustre to hair and makes soft and dark.
- Baldness can be controlled by using Rogan Jara-rech and Rogan Baiza Murg.
- Lice of hair can be removed by using "Zarbin".

Herbal Cosmetics from the Ancient Texts

FOR HAIR CARE

Important uses of oil

नित्यं स्नेहार्द्र शिरसः शिरःशूलं न जायते।
न खालित्यं न पालित्यं न केशाः प्रपतन्तिच।।
बलं शिरः कपलानां विशेषणाभिवर्धते।
दृढमूलाश्च दीर्घाश्च कृष्णाः केशा भवन्ति च।। (च.सू. 4/81-83)

Regular application (massage) of oil on the scalp relieves one from headaches, prevents baldness, greying of hair, and hairfall.

It is also helpful in improving power tone of the head and rest of the body. The hair roots will become firm, resulting in long and black hair. **(Charaka Sutra)**

❖❖❖

केश प्रसाधनी केश्या रजोजन्तुमलापहा। (सु.चि. 24/29)

Regular hair care in the form of cleaning and combing not only keeps hair in sound health, but also frees it from extraneous dirt and lice. **(Sushruta Chikitsa)**

❖❖❖

शिरोगतांस्तथा रोगा झूछरोऽभ्यंगोऽपकर्षति ।
केशानां मार्दवं दैर्घ्य बहूत्वं स्निग्धकृष्णताम् ।।
करोति शिरस्तृप्ति सुत्वक्रमपि चाननम् ।
सन्तर्पणं चेन्द्रियाणां शिरसः प्रतिपूरणम् ।। (सु.चि. 24/25-26)

An oil massage on the head not only helps the hair grow strong, dark, soft and shiny, it also relieves afflictions that can originate in the head. It helps to keep the mind cool and contented and also adds a glow of radiance to the face. Oil massage also enlivens the vital organs and rejuvenates the brain.

(Sushruta Chikitsa)

❖◆❖

Etiopathology of Alopecia (Baldness)

रोमकूपानुगं पित्तं वातेन सह मुर्च्छितम् ।
प्रॅच्यावयति रोमाणि ततः श्लेष्मा सशोणितः ।।
रूणभ्दि रोगकूपांस्तु ततोन्येषामसम्भवः ।
तदिन्द्रलुप्तं खालित्यं रूज्येति च विभाव्यते ।। (सु.चि. 23/32-33)

Deranged pitta in hair follicle along with deranged vata dosha acts upon its tip as well as on the root and destroys it as a result of which hair loss occurs.

Deranged pitta in turn leads to derangement of rakta dhatu and kapha dosha. The kapha dosha loses its normal consistency and becomes more viscous and sticky and as a result of this changes the viscid kapha along with rakta dosha blocking the opening of Romakupa (pores of hair). So further growth of hair is inhibited.

(Sushruta Chikitsa)

❖◆❖

कासीसं नक्तमालस्य पल्लवांश्चैव संहरेत् ।
कपित्थरसपिष्टानि रोमसंजननं परम् ।। (सु.चि. 1/103)

Sulphate of iron i.e. Kasisa ($FeSO_4 \cdot 7H_2O$) and tender Karanja leaves pasted with expressed juice of Kapittha should be applied to the spot where the growth of hair (Lomotpatti) is desired i.e. regeneration.

(Sushruta Chikitsa)

❖◆❖

हस्तिदन्तमसीं कृत्वा मुख्यं चैव रसांजनम् ।
रोमाण्येतेन जायन्ते लेपात्पाणितलेष्वपि ।। (सु.चि. 1/105)

Hasthi danta mashi (burnt ash of ivory) and Rasanjan when mixed with goat milk and applied on the scalp, effects regeneration of hair within 7 days. **(Sushruta Chikitsa)**

❖❖❖

शंशचूर्णस्य भागौ दूवौ हरतालं च भागिकम् ।
शुक्तेन सह पिष्टानि लोमशातनमुत्तमम् ।। (सु.चि. 1/105)

One part of shankha powder and two parts of Hartal powder mixed with Shukti and applied on hair root is best for removal of unwanted hair on the body. **(Sushruta Chikitsa)**

क्रोधशोकश्रमकृतः शरीरोष्मा शिरोगतः ।
पित्तं च केशान् पचति वालितं तेन जायते ।। (सु.चि. 13/36)

The pitta and ushna (internal heat) generated due to anger, grief and stress strike at the head (or hair root) resulting in premature greying of hair. **(Sushruta Chikitsa)**

10. Eye Care

The eyes are the mirror of health and the most expressive features of the face. Beautiful, bright eyes are a part of 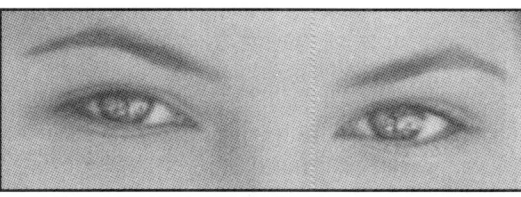 radiant health and the best asset one can have. They give a wonderful effect to one's personality. Dull and lustreless eyes are an indication of ill health and depressed state of mind. During sickness, the eyes are the first to tell their story of pain.

Dull Eyes

The main causes of dull and lustreless eyes are physical and mental strain resulting from overwork, worry, fear and anxiety, faulty diet and improper blood and nerve supply. Watching too much television, films, excessive reading, reading either in dim or bright light leads to physical strain on the eyes. Dull eyes are a general symptom of a general toxaemic condition of the body, mainly due to excessive intake of starch, sugar and protein. The muscles and blood vessels surrounding the eyes share in the clogging process taking place due to improper metabolism by imbalanced and highly concentrated diet.

Natural Care

The first important factor in restoring normal health and sparkle to the eyes is to loosen the strained and contracted muscles surrounding them. This can be achieved through the eye muscle and neck exercises as mentioned below:

Eye exercise

- Keep the head still and relaxed, gently move the eyes up and down six times. Repeat the same movement two or three times after a rest of two or three seconds in between.
- Move the eyes six times from side to side, as far as possible, without any force or effort. Repeat two or three times.
- Move the eyes gently and slowly around in a circle, and then move them low in the reverse direction. Do this four times in all. Rest for two or three seconds and repeat the movement two or three times, using minimum effort.

Neck exercise

- Rotate the neck in circles and semi-circles.
- Move the shoulders anti-clockwise briskly, drawing them up as far as possible several times.
- Allow the head to droop forward and backward as far as possible several times. These exercises help to loosen up the contracted neck muscles, which may restrict blood supply to the head.

Palming

Sit in a comfortable position in an armchair and relax with your eyes closed. Cover the eyes with the palms, right palm over the right eye and left palm over the left eye. Do not press on the eyes. Then, with your eyes completely covered in this manner, allow your elbows to drop on your knees, keeping the knees fairly close together. With eyes closed thus, try to imagine blankness, which grows blacker and blacker. Palming reduces strain and relaxes the eyes and its surrounding tissues.

Diet

Diet is of utmost importance for the health and beauty of the eyes. A healthy diet of milk, butter, fruits, green vegetables and proteins should be taken for proper care of the eyes. Natural, uncooked foods are the best diet. These include fresh fruits, green vegetables, nuts, dry fruits, and dairy products. Cereals are also necessary, but they should be consumed sparingly.

Genuine whole meal bread is the best and most suitable. Denatured foods like white flour, white sugar and all products made from them, tea and coffee, together with meat and fish soon play havoc with the digestion and the body. They should, therefore, be avoided as far as possible. Constipating or wind-forming foods, alcohol and other intoxicating substances are also harmful and should be avoided.

Vitamin A

Each of the essential nutrients needed by the body plays some part in the health and beauty of the eyes. The effect of vitamin A upon the eyes is, however, most pronounced. For normal and healthy eyes, a liberal amount of vitamin A must be continuously supplemented with the food. The valuable sources of this vitamin are cod liver oil, whole milk, curds, butter, egg yolk, pumpkin, carrot, green leafy vegetables, tomato, mango, papaya, orange and melon.

Natural Aids

Amongst the various natural substances, the use of castor oil is highly beneficial for the eyes. This causes increased lachrymation of the eyes for a while, but leaves the eyes clean and cool. Regular massage on the scalp with castor oil decreases eye strain.

Ayurvedic Aid

Triphala, an ayurvedic preparation consisting of Emblic myrobalan (Amla), Chebulic myrobalan (Harad), and Belleric myrobalan (Bahara), is considered beneficial for long eyelashes and sparkling eyes. A teaspoon of this preparation should be soaked overnight in a cup of water. It should be poured through a muslin cloth and the eyes should be dabbed in it for a minute. Dust, smoke, draughts of cold or hot winds, bright objects are all harmful to the eyes and should be avoided. The eyes should also be kept protected from sunlight, and it is advisable to wear sunglasses outdoors.

Eye Cream for Dark Circles Under the Eyes

Preparation
- 1 tablespoon lanolin.
- 1½ tablespoons almond oil.
- 1 teaspoon soyabean flour.
- 2 teaspoons cold water.

Application

Melt lanolin on medium heat. Add almond oil to it. Remove the ensuing thick paste from heat. Add soyabean powder and cold water to it and stir for 10 minutes. Do not mix fragrance while preparing the eye cream. It might affect the eyes. Using eye cream is useful if there are circles or dark spots beneath the eyes.

Care of the Skin Around the Eyes

The skin around the eyes is more prone to wear and tear, caused by the mechanical action of squinting and blinking. The often puffy look can be attributed to retention of oil by the skin. As a result of ageing, the muscle tone around the eye weakens and the skin loses its elasticity, resulting in the formation of crow's feet and bags under the eyes.

To slow down the ageing process you need to follow a few do's and don'ts:

- Get enough sleep.
- Don't rub your eyes. Rubbing stretches the thin eye skin and encourages bags.
- Use a moisturiser—heavy on the eyelid, lighter on the under-eye—night and day.
- Eye exercises done regularly increase blood flow to the eye.

Haldi and Tulsi can fight Cataract

Cataract is responsible for the maximum number of visually impaired persons in the country today (nearby 12 million people suffering from cataract). Scientific experiment at AIIMS, New Delhi have revealed that a combination of Tulsi and Haldi extracts can control cataract formation. This formulation is patented and its eye drop will be available soon. This will stop oxidative stress of eyes which leads to cataract formation. Haldi and Tulsi can delay and even prevent or stop formation of insoluble proteins that obstruct vision.

Keeping an Eye for Cure

Recent findings to check age-related blindness eg. Cataract is to make use of a magic plant *Withania Somnifera* (Ashwagandha). Researchers say by regular intake of extract of this plant or its root powder delay the cataract formation by 45%.

●●

11. Essential Oil

Cleopatra, Aphrodite, Helen of Troy, King Tut and Jesus benefited from the beauty, health and anti-ageing properties in pure plant oils. "Oil free" was a term unheard of in those days.

We have been misled, folks! Contrary to popular beliefs, oils are essential for your skin's health. In *Encyclopaedia of Anti-ageing Remedies*, John Heinemann writes about how essential fatty acids or EFAs are good for the health of the skin. Our bodies cannot produce them. They come from the diet or supplements. He says, "The two EFAs are omega-3 (alpha-linolenic acid) and omega-6 (linoleic acid). Four of the very best sources of such omega-3 fatty acid are cod liver oil (1 tbsp daily), and evening primrose oil (4 capsules daily)."

We have come to believe that oils clog the skin and cause skin eruptions. Creamy chemical-laden products do just that. But a body that is lacking the proper oils has the side effects of dry, parched, ageing skin. Take all the fats and oils out of your diet and out of your skin care products and you will go from being a plump juicy grape to a dried-up old raisin long before your time.

Avocado Oil: It is a wonderful, non-irritating oil that is used as a base for all blended body oils. Each ounce is packed with many active ingredients like vitamin A (20,000 IU), vitamin D (40,000 IU) and vitamin E (300 IU).

Carrot Oil: It has tons of vitamins and is a super skin food. It is also non-irritating, so you can use it topically.

Evening Primrose Oil: It is a super-powered, super beauty oil packed with essential fatty acids. Use it topically and take it internally.

Olive Oil: It contains essential fatty acids and is a good, non-irritating base oil. It is one of the best oils you can take internally.

Wheat Germ Oil: It is packed with vitamin E and essential fatty acids, and is also a good, non-irritating base oil.

Sun Flower Oil: It has lots of essential fatty acids and is virtually non-irritating.

The Blending of Oils

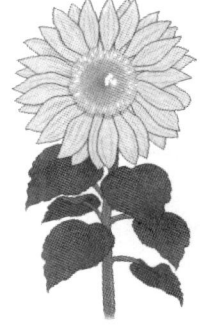

The beauty of blending your own oils is that you get to customise them to your own special needs and liking. You'll find that blending your own oils is also simple, and liberating. You'll want to use a six-ounce jar for blending your oils. The vitamins you'll use come in gel caps. You can stick them with a pin or snip them with a pair of scissors and squeeze the vitamins into the jar. Put the lid on and handshake vigorously. Below is the formula.

The Glow Oil Recipe
- ◆ Pour four ounces of a base oil (usually avocado because of its rich, active ingredients) into a six-ounce container or jar.
- ◆ Add 500 mg each of vitamins A, D, and E.
- ◆ As a finishing touch, add 2,000 mg of evening primrose oil.

You can purchase all the above oils and vitamins at your local health food store. Try apricot kernel oil as an even lighter base and add some of your essential oils, lavender, rose or jasmine for a flowery scent if you like. Make sure you include the vitamins listed in the above recipe.

You don't need to use much of any oil, just a few drops on each part of your body. It is light and absorbed easily into your skin. It leaves absolutely no oily or greasy residue.

Scented Baths

15-20 drops ($^1/_8$ dram) essential oil or oil blend.

¾ dram carrier oil.

1½-3 ounces Epsom salt.

Be certain that it is mixed thoroughly, as the oil may have a tendency to form into clumps in the salt. Even distribution is required. Also note that this will make several baths. It only takes 1½ to 2 teaspoons of mixture for an entire bath. While there are different preferred methods for preparing the aromatic baths, two of them emerge as the easiest and least complicated in the preparatory stages. One is to introduce the essential oil or oil blend into a small amount of Epsom salts, and to dissolve the salts into a tub of hot or warm water. Some take the trouble to add colour and fixatives to the mixture to produce something comparable to the commercially available bath salts. Unless the intention is to market the end product, this is really unnecessary. In fact, the salts can be prepared just minutes prior to the time of use.

If the essential oil blend contains ingredients that may act as irritants, you may be able to still utilise their virtuous properties if you increase the amount of Epsom salt and introduce a carrier oil to dilute the oil blend. However, if you are not certain that you can eliminate the negative effects of the irritants, it may be wiser to choose another method of administering the remedy altogether.

Another method of creating an aromatic bath is to introduce the essential oil blend directly into the bath water. Although this is a viable way to prepare a bath quickly, it is not the choice method for optimum effectiveness. Because oil and water do not truly mix, it is easier to get an even distribution of the fragrance if a moment is taken to mix the essential oil blend with the bath salts before adding it to the water.

Like heated massage oil, the warmth of the freshly drawn bath serves to open the pores of the skin. Thus, in addition to the benefits of inhalation while immersed in the scented water, the individual is actually taking in the healing properties of the essential blend through the skin. Aromatic baths are used in many of the available applications of the fragrance arts. They can be directed toward ritual, toward healing mind, body, and spirit, or as a lavish way of pampering oneself to beauty and elegance.

Fragrant Herbal Bath

Humulus lupulus	450g
Thymus serpyllum	25g
Salvia officinalis	25g
Lavender	25g

Put the ingradients into a muslin bag and tie securely. Hang the bag from the hot tap while the bath is running, so that the hot water passes through it, extracting the natural oils and fragrance of the herbs. This bath will help relax tired muscles and relieve rheumatism.

A Gift from Heaven

In antiquity, honey was regarded as a gift from the heavens and it was widely believed that it simply rained from the sky and was collected by bees. It was rightly called "Saliva from the Stars". Aromatic beauty food routine is not complete without the use of honey in their preparation.

12. Preparing Herbal Cosmetics at Home

Most herbal remedies won't require more than the supplies that you normally find in your kitchen. However, it is recommended that you try to accumulate a separate set of measuring and stirring tools, bowls, grinders, pots, and more to be set aside just for making herbal blends and treatments.

Cooking Tips

Be sure that all of your cookware for making herbal remedies is made of non-reactive materials such as glass, enamel, or stainless steel, and not reactive metals such as copper or aluminium.

Here is a list of basic provisions:

- All-purpose mixing bowls in a variety of sizes.
- Coffee grinder.
- Cutting board.
- Double boiler.
- Funnels.
- Glass eyedropper.
- Grater.
- Heavy-duty plastic zip-seal storage bags.
- Ice cube trays.
- Jars with screw-top lids, preferably of tinted glass.
- Kitchen or garden shears.
- Kitchen scale.
- Labels and marking pens.
- Measuring cups with metric and imperial measurements.

- Measuring spoons.
- Mortar and pestle.
- Multispeed blender or food processor.
- Non-reactive pots and saucepans with lids.
- Sieves: fine-mesh cheesecloth, unbleached muslin, paper coffee filters, nylon or stainless steel mesh.
- Utensils: paring knife, ladle, wooden mallet, vegetable peeler, rolling pin, spatula, wooden spoons, whisk.

Instructions

- Your nose is the best indicator of the freshness of oil or any other substance useful in cosmetics and you should discard any rancid oil/substance distinguishable by sour, foul odour.
- To prevent spoilage, oils should be stored in containers that shield them as much as possible from light and air.
- To increase the shelf life of your hand-made cosmetics make sure that the utensils and workspace used to make them are clean and sterile. Use utensils that are reserved exclusively for making cosmetics and wash them properly and strengthen them by placing them in a pot of boiling water for 15 minutes.
- Make your cosmetics in small batches and pour them into clean pump dispensers and bottles with flip-top lids. Refrigerate them separately from food in a crisper.
- Always refrain from dipping your fingers into your products to avoid transmission of harmful bacteria into them. Use a plastic cosmetic spatula or a popsicle stick to dispense cream from non-pump jar.

Weights and Measures

The emulsion and other liquid herbal cosmetic recipes described in the book are stated in teaspoon or tablespoon measures. A conversion table on grams vs. spoonful is given below, so that one can prepare these recipes in required quantity, as the shelf-life of these natural cosmetics is very short.

Item/Ingredient	One Teaspoon	One Table Spoonful
Water/Oil	4 Grams	14 Grams
Glycerin (Vegetable Origin)	6 Grams	16 Grams
Almond Oil and Other Oils	4 Grams	12 Grams
Butter/Other Solids	4 Grams	12 Grams
Borax (Tankan)	3 Grams	11 Grams

60 drops = 1 teaspoon (5 ml)
3 teaspoons = 1 tablespoon
1 oz = 28.3 grams

Note: The same volume of different ingredients weighs differently and records are made in a notebook to maintain the uniformity of the product.

Herbal Cosmetics Ingredients—Guide

Acacia shrub or tree (Acacia senegal)
Also known as: Gum-arabic tree.
Parts used: Gummy substance secreted from the bark.
Properties: Gum acacia is soluble in water, contains magnesium and potassium; the gum can be used with other cover material or wrap-inflamed tissues.

Almond, sweet (Prunus dulcis var. dulcis)
Parts used: Nut or seed, powder, oil pressed from the seed.
Properties: Demulcent, emollient, nutritive (a source of iron, calcium, potassium, copper, zinc, vitamin E, biotin, plus 18 of the 20 amino acids needed for healthy growth), skin softener; often used in body oils and lotions.

Valerian (Valeriana officinalis)
Parts used: Root or rhizome.
Properties: A natural relaxant, calming, sedative, mild pain reliever.

Anti-oxidant vitamins (A, C, E) and minerals (Cu, Zn, Se)
Keep the skin and its texture intact and protect it from oxidative processes that takes place on exposure e.g. sun-rays and environmental pollutions. To combat it one should eat fresh coloured vegetable and fruits.

Baking soda (Sodium bicarbonate)

Parts used: Powder.

Properties: Alkaline, skin conditioner; soothes minor skin irritations, including bee stings and itching.

Beeswax

Properties: Obtained from the honeycomb of honeybees; holds fatty oils in emulsion in moisturising creams and lotions; natural beeswax is dark yellow.

Benzoin (Styrax benzoin)

Also known as: Gum benzoin.
Parts used: Tree resin, tincture of benzoin.
Properties: Antiseptic and astringent; used to heal inflamed, irritated, and cracked skin bothered by the environment; improves skin elasticity; cosmetic fixative and preservative of fats.

Borax (Sodium borate)

Parts used: White, crystalline, mineral powder.
Properties: Antiseptic, emulsifier, and buffering agent for moisturisers, scrubs, bath salts.

Burdock (Arctium lappa)

Parts used: Crushed seeds (fruits) inside sticky burs, root, and leaves.
Properties: Adaptogen, demulcent, diaphoretic, diuretic, bitter; cleanses body system to relieve skin problems; useful as an aid in treatments of arthritis; contains B-vitamins, iron and sulphur.
Caution: Not recommended for use during pregancy or by nursing mothers.

Carrot (Daucus carota var. sativa)

Parts used: Whole herb, mashed; seeds and root; seed oil.
Properties: Rich in Beta carotene and antioxidant vitamins and minerals; diuretic, carminative, stimulant; a 10 percent dilution of the seed oil can be used to prevent scar formation and improve skin texture. It is a potent source of Vitamin A.

Castor oil

Properties: A heavy, protective, soothing oil; laxative; helps to seal in moisture in skin preparations. It is anti-rheumatic also.

Cayenne pepper (Capsicum annuum)

Also known as: Chile pepper.
Parts used: Fruit, ripe and dried.
Properties: Contains capsaicin, a powerful local stimulant and rubefacient that increases the flow of blood and oxygenation of body cells, produces natural warmth, and functions as an antiseptic; can be prepared as a tincture to treat cold hands and feet.

Cedar, red (Thuja plicata)

Parts used: Fan-like beaches of young trees.
Properties: Antifungal and antibacterial; stimulates immune response; leaves are often used for incense; can be prepared as a tincture to treat nail fungus.

Cedar, white (Thuja occidentalis)

Also known as: Arborvitae.
Parts used: New growth, leafy, terminal twigs.
Properties: Antibacterial, antiviral, diuretic, nervine; can be used to treat warts, skin fungus, and itchy skin disorders.
Caution: Not recommended for use during pregnancy or by nursing mothers.

Cocoa butter

Properties: The fat is used in making ointments and cosmetic creams; has a chocolate aroma.

Coconut butter and oil

Properties: Coconut oil comes from the coconut palm (cocos nucifera). Copra, coconut meat, is called coconut butter. Coconut oil and butter are skin softeners; often used in emollient ointments and creams.

Corn (Zea mays)

Parts used: Cornmeal, cornstarch, corn oil, corn silk.

Properties: Cornmeal can be used as a mild abrasive; corn starch can be used as a thickener; corn oil can be used as an emollient for nails and skin; corn silk, the pistils of the flowers, can be used as a diuretic when taken as tea.

Flax (Linum ustitatissimum)
Also known as: Linseed.
Parts used: Seeds, oil from seeds.
Properties: Emollient, demulcent; richer in omega-3 oils (or omega-3 acids) than fish; crushed seeds offer healing mucilage for poultices to treat abscesses and boils by reducing irritation, pain, and inflammation.

Garlic (Allium sativum)
Parts used: Bulb, fresh cloves, juice.
Properties: Antiseptic, antibiotic, anti-viral, anti-allergy, aphrodisiac, anti-amoebic, anti-coagulant, detoxifier, carminative, diaphoretic, and stimulant; may protect the heart and nervous system, enhance the body's immune system, decrease the side effects of drug therapies for cancer. The therapeutically active ingredient in garlic is the smelly allicin. Garlic also contains amino acids, selenium, sulphur, B-vitamins, and minerals.
Caution: Fresh garlic juice on the skin can cause blistering in delicate persons.

Ginger (Zingiber officinale)
Parts used: Dried rhizome, oil, and powder.
Properties: Anti-inflammatory, circulatory stimulant, and antiseptic; controls nausea; drinking ginger tea will bring blood to the surface and warm cold hands and feet. Apart from it, it is antiviral agent.

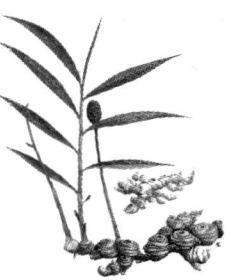

Ginkgo (Ginkgo biloba)
Parts used: Leaves, seeds.
Properties: Gingko leaves are a circulatory stimulant. They increase blood flow to the brain, enhance energy, and improve peripheral circulation to the hands and feet, and more.

Henna (Lawsonia inermis, L.alba)
Parts used: Powdered leaves, flowers.

Properties: As a dye for the skin or nails, tinting the hair anti-fungal, antiseptic.

Honey

Properties: Emollient, humectants, antiseptic, and bacteriostatic; helps skin retain moisture; can be applied to a wound as a cooling analgesic.

Jojoba (Simmondisa chinensis)

Parts used: Seeds, extract of the seeds.

Properties: Jojoba extract is an unusual wax ester with antioxidant, anti-microbial, anti-inflammatory, and light emollient properties. It is similar in chemistry to human sebum, the skin's natural restorative fluid. Can help to maintain the suppleness of the skin; conditions and softens skin, hair, and scalp; can aid the healing of wounds; can be used alone or as a base for ointments and creams for dry, chapped skin, as a cuticle and nail conditioner, and with aloe for minor burns and sunburn. Jojoba has few impurities; contains no resins, tars, or alkaloids; and is non-toxic and non-allergenic.

Kaolin clay

Properties: Soft, white clay that draws oils and impurities from the skin.

Lavender (Lavandula spp.)

Parts used: Flowers, essential oil.

Properties: Pleasant antiseptic, antidepressive, and antimicrobial; calming effect to relieve stress; essential oil can be used externally for aching muscles and to help prevent scarring.

Caution: Avoid during first trimester of pregnancy; not recommended for those with very low blood pressure.

Lemon (Citrus limon)

Parts used: Juice, pulp, rind, essential oil.

Properties: Astringent, bleaching, disinfectant; scent is stimulating and refreshing; anti-inflammatory.

Caution: Do not use essential oil in strong sunlight or on sensitive skin.

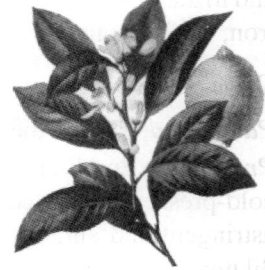

Lemon grass (Cymbopogon citratus)

Parts used: Grass, essential oil.

Properties: Refreshing, lemon-like tonic; antiseptic, antidepressant, and astringent.

Caution: Avoid during pregnancy, and do not use on sensitive skin.

Lime (Tilia spp)

Also known as: Linden tree.

Parts used: Flowers, essential oil.

Properties: Nervine, diuretic, tonic; reduces nervous tension; calming; can be a soothing and softening agent in skin-care products.

Milk, butter and cream

Properties: Can be used as a skin cleanser and as emollient in creams and lotions.

Mint (Mentha spicata)

Parts used: Leaves, essential oil.

Properties: Stimulant, carminative, antispasmodic, diaphoretic; relieves stomach complaints; can be used for flavouring.

Myrrh (Commiphora molmol)

Parts used: Gum resin, volatile oil.

Properties: Anti-fungal, anti-bacterial, anti-viral agent; antiseptic, cooling and tonic; good for wounds that refuse to heal, boils and abscesses.

Oats, oat straw (Avena sativa)

Parts used: Oatmeal or oat bran, seeds, or grains.

Properties: Exfoliant and emollient for chapped hands, eczema, and irritated, dry, or itching skin; source of vitamin E, proteins, zinc, iron, and manganese.

Olive (Olea europaea)

Parts used: Oil of the fruit, leaves.

Properties: Emollient, demulcent, laxative, source of linoleic acid; cold-pressed oil is used in salves for muscle pains; leaves in tea are astringent and antiseptic; may lower blood sugar in diabetes and dilate coronary arteries to improve blood circulation.

Onion (Allium cepa)

Parts used: Bulb.

Properties: Antiseptic, aphrodisiac, antibacterial, anti-inflammatory, and diuretic; rich in vitamin B1, B2, and C; stimulates the heart and reduces blood sugar.

Orange (Citrus aurantium)

Parts used: Fruit, flowers, rind.

Properties: Essential oil of sweet orange blossoms, called neroli, has antiseptic, anti-depressant, and tonic properties and is a perfect choice for sensitive skin. Essential oil of the leaves and young shoots of orange plant, called oil of petit grain, is natural skin toner and stimulant but may be a bit harsh for sensitive skin.

Papaya (Carica papaya)

Parts used: Fruit, juice, leaves.

Properties: Juice and fruit of the fresh plant can be used for wounds that refuse to heal and to remove freckles; contains papain, an enzyme that can improve digestion of proteins; leaves may be used as a substitute for soap.

Paraffin (Petroselinum cripsum)

Parts used: Leaves, stems.

Properties: Anti-microbial, cleansing, and diuretic; rich in potassium, calcium, and silica; may strengthen nails and skin; reduces smell of garlic and onions on breath and hands.

Caution: Not recommended in large doses during pregnancy or for those with kidney inflammation.

Pineapple (Ananas comosus)

Parts used: Juice, fruit.

Properties: Anti-inflammatory; gargle for sore throat.

Raspberry (Rubus idaeus)

Parts used: Fruit, leaves.

Properties: Astringent and stimulant; can be used as a wash for wounds and external skin ulcers.

Rose, otto of (Rosa damascene)

Parts used: Essential oil from the flower.

Properties: Astringent, tonic, antiseptic, anti-inflammatory; promotes the formation of new skin cells; especially useful for dry, sensitive, ageing skin.

Caution: Limited use during pregnancy.

Rosemary (Rosmarinus officinalis)

Parts used: Leaves and stems.

Properties: Antispasmodic, rubefacient, and fragrant stimulant; can be used in a liniment to treat painful joints and stiff muscles. In ancient times, rosemary had a reputation for strengthening the memory.

Sage (Salvia officinalis)

Parts used: Leaves, whole herb.

Properties: Astringent and stimulant; used to treat joint pain.

Caution: Not recommended in large doses during pregnancy or by those with high blood pressure or epilepsy.

Sea salt

Properties: Rich in minerals; circulatory stimulant in a scrub; can remove dead surface skin cells and dirt.

Caution: May burn broken skin.

Sea weed (Laminaria digitata)

Also known as: Kelp.

Parts used: Seaweed flakes and powder.

Properties: Emollient; rich in vitamins and minerals.

Shea butter (Botyrospermum parkii)

Also known as: Karite butter.

Properties: Can be added to moisturisers for the reduction of wrinkles and to creams for sore muscles, rheumatism, burns, and light wounds; antioxidant with a high linoleum acid content; good for dry or irritable skin, sunburn, chapping; offers skin protection against ultraviolet rays; increases capillary circulation; good for sensitive skin.

Tea tree (Melaleuca alternifolia)

Parts used: Essential oil.

Properties: Antifungal, anti-bacterial, tissue cleanser; a 10% solution of the essential oil is a safe external antiseptic for skin diseases, fungal infections, and wounds.

Vitamin E oil

Also known as: Natural d-alpha tocopherol (other forms are synthetic).

Properties: A natural preservative; discourages scarring, encourages healing of wounds.

Yoghurt

Properties: Mildly astringent; rich in B-complex vitamins; contains helpful bacteria that act to restore normal chemical balance to the intestines and aid the body's digestive system.

Aloe (Aloe-vera)

Parts used: Gel from the succulent leaves; some suppliers sell aloe "juice" which does not have the same healing properties as the gel.

Properties: Demulcent, antibacterial, antibiotic, source of allantoin; useful for healing cuts and wounds, as an analgesic for mild pain, and for soothing sunburn.

Caution: Not recommended for use during pregnancy.

Medicinal uses of Aloe-vera

1. Dissolved in water of roses it is used in various eye troubles.
2. The fresh juice of leaves is useful in fever, spleen and liver diseases and enlarged lymphatic glands.
3. Aloe gel is used with milk in dysentry and kidney infection.
4. Aloes is used for colitis, diarrhoea and digestive trouble.
5. A piece of the pulp which is peeled to the size of ½ a finger is inserted into the rectum in haemorrhoids and bleeding piles.
6. Peptic and duodenal ulcers can be cured by taking one pint blended gel at regular interval daily.
7. In cases of enlarged spleen juice of the leaf with powdered turmeric is given.
8. In case of chronic fissures and ulcers around the rectum, aloe is largely used both internally and externally.
9. It is anthelmintic and good medicine for kids' intestinal worms.

13. Aroma Therapy

Aromatherapy, which can be regarded as recent branch of Phytotherapy (a treatment with herb/plant products), here concerns the use of essential oils for their healing properties. However, as claimed, aromatherapy is recent discovery but it is more correct to say it as rediscovery. We know that our ancestors used essential oils to embalm their dead (due to their antiseptic properties), to render putrefied substances more tolerable and as food preservatives and further more as perfume. All essential oils or essences can be divided into three classes: (a) **Terpenic** (b) **Oxygenated** and (c) **Sulphurized**. All have curative, antiseptic and anti-bacterial properties and, above all, different chemical structures.

Recent research now showed that essences perform a specific antibiotic action and produce no secondary effects whatsoever on the organic functioning of the body, so, wider use e.g. essence of *thyme* has great antiseptic power than hydrogen peroxide and guaicol due to its thymol content.

A water solution of thyme kills the typhus bacillus in two minutes, streptocoecus in four minutes and T.B. bacillus in one hour. Similarly, essence of lemon kills the meningitis bacillus in a quarter of an hour and staphylococeus and pneumococeus in one hour.

Cure with Sweet Smelling Compounds

It is interesting to recall that in olden days people sprinkled themselves with the essence of rosemary, thyme, sage and other fragrant plants as a protection against contagious diseases during epidemics. The good sense of this practice is today fully endorsed, as is proved by our own current use of *atomized sprays* comprising a mixture of essences with phenolic content which can easily sterilize a room full of bacilli. If such procedures are adopted in hospitals and operating theatres, almost total asepsis could be achieved.

Essences, however, are not only effective because of their bacterial action. There is much evidence to show that their healing effect is, in fact, obtained by means of a range of activities.

Essences can be divided according to these activities: antispasmodic or spasmolytic, stimulatory, antifermentative and hormonal. In this connection, it is remarkable how the traditional use of certain plants has now been justified by qualitative analyses of their essences.

It has been proved that many plants, for example, produce substances with hormonal qualities similar to the female ovarian hormones and, therefore, behave in the same way. Sage, hops, willow and liquorice have long been popular remedies to increase the milk flow of a nursing mother or to correct and stabilize the menstrual flow, and science has now confirmed their efficacy and revealed the reasons for it. There are probably many other types of plant that produce such hormones, or others that are akin to them. It is important, therefore, that these valuable natural resources should be discovered, classified and used under strict medical control to avoid dependence on ill-tolerated *synthetic* preparations.

Many people have personal experience of the antiputrefactive and antifermentive uses of certain essential oil-producing plants such as fennel, anise and coriander, which are especially effective remedies against such complaints as gastritis and colitis.

In this broad survey of the efficacy of essential oils, one indirect consequence seems worth mentioning. Many of these oils are used in the cosmetic and perfume industries. The cosmetic expert, therefore, must work closely with someone who has knowledge of aromatherapy.

●●

14. Quick Herbal Remedies

Problem	Herbal Remedy
Burning of feet and palms	A poultice made from henna plant leaves + vinegar is very effective. (without vinegar is also effective). The juice of eclipta alba (bhringraj) leaves can also be applied. Sandalwood oil can be applied.
Corn	Apply the milky juice of papaya fruit daily till it becomes soft.
Cracking of the soles of palms/feet	Pure til oil or ghee should be applied daily at bedtime. Cashew nut oil can also be used. Pinda oil: medicated oil with beeswax base is the ideal application.
Dandruff	Emulsion made with sandalwood oil and lemon juice is very effective. 1 part of sandalwood oil should be mixed with three parts of lemon juice.
Dark circles below eyes	Regular application of the following removes these ugly circles gradually. Fresh tomato juice. Paste of raw potato. Pack of almond. Turmeric + lime juice. Fresh cucumber juice + honey.
For complexion	A paste prepared from the thorny skin of the silk-cotton tree, with milk can be applied to the skin of the face. It brings lustre to the face.
Greying hair	Neeli bhringa amlaki oil's regular application successfully prevents hair greying.
Head lice	Prepare the paste of bitter almonds by adding a little water and apply. The paste made of finely powdered seeds of custard apple (sharifa) with water should be applied at bedtime and the head well covered with cloth.

Problem	Herbal Remedy
Herpes	The emulsion of the oil expressed from pongamia pinnata (karanja) made with lemon juice is very effective in healing.
Natural sunscreen	Application of castor oil (Dabur) before going out on a sunny day prevents sunburns and works like a herbal sunscreen.
Natural hair colourants	Henna, manjista, tea leaves, coffee powder, jatamamsi.
Natural perfumes	Japa, jasmine, kachura.
Prickly heat	The paste made from equal parts of sandalwood, coriander seeds, tubercles of nut grass (mustaka), roots of khuskhus grass powdered together and mixed with rosewater applied on the body gives immediate relief.
Rough, dry, coarse skin	Applying the powder of the seeds of fenugreek (methi) with a little water (make paste) makes the skin smooth.
Spots and freckles on the skin	Apply cottonseed oil daily. It clears spots on the skin.
Skin burn	1. Apply two teaspoons tomato juice and 4 tablespoons of buttermilk. Leave on the face and wash after half an hour. 2. Mix olive oil with equal quantity of vinegar and apply one hour before you bathe.
Thin hair (hairfall)	Bhringraj hair oil improves hair growth.
Warts	Pure oil of cashew nut (kaju) should be applied over the warts, till they fall off. Kasisadi oil, an ayurvedic medicated oil, can be applied on corns and warts, regularly— these will become soft and ultimately fall off.
Whitlow	The paste of garlic and black pepper may be applied over the affected nail matrix. It relieves pain.
Wrinkles over face	Pack made of egg yolk and one spoon of honey reduces wrinkles.

Glossary
Herbal Cosmetics Available in the Market

Problem	Herbal cosmetics	Manufacturing company
Acne	Acne-n-pimple cream (external use)	Ayurvedic Concepts
	Blood purifier	Himalaya-Ayur Concepts
	Shamint (to remove excess oil)	Himalaya-Ayur concepts
	Shazeema (medicated soap for acne)	Shahnaz Hussain
	Shaclear (for drying pimples)	Shahnaz Hussain
		Shahnaz Hussain
Anti-wrinkle creams	Naturene	Naturene
	Sunscreen	Synergie
	Flawless cream	Nature's Way
Blemishes (pimple or other marks)	Gentle exfoliating scrub	Himalaya
	Beauty grains	Shahnaz Hussain
	Shabeen	Shahnaz Hussain
	Banjara's skin food	Banjara
Cleaning	Gentle cleaning milk	Synergie
	Gentle face wash	Synergie
	Gentle face wash cream	Ayurvedic Concepts
	Gentle face scrub	Ayurvedic Concepts
	Gentle exfoliating scrub	Ayurvedic Concepts
	Deep cleaning face mask	Synergie
	Deep cleaning lotion	Himalaya/Ayurvedic Concepts
Dry skin	Moisturising lotion for dry skin	Ayurvedic Concepts
	Rich moisturising Lotion	Ayurvedic Concepts
	Revitalising cream	Ayurvedic Concepts
	Sha-dew	Shahnaz Hussain
	Sha-glow	Shahnaz Hussain
Dandruff	Anti-dandruff hair cleanser	Himalaya
	Anti-dandruff hair vitaliser	Himalaya
	Shanel	Shahnaz Hussain
	Sha-hair (henna powder for dandruff)	Shahnaz Hussain

Dark circles under eye	Under eye gel	Synergie
Fairness	Shahnaz Shafair Godrej Fairglow soap	Shahnaz Godrej
For promotion of complexion	Kumkumadi Lepam Vicco-turmeric Swaroop Lep	Imcops Vicco Laboratories Amrutha
Hair falling Best cure for hair fall is to take a table spoon of almond oil, one teaspoon of castor oil, 5 to 6 drops of lavender oil and 2 drops of rosemary oil and massage into hair.	Revitalising hair nutrient oil Sha tone oil Sha locks lotion Original Brahmi oil lotion Mahabhring raj oil. Nourishing hair cleaner shampoo	Himalaya Shahnaz Hussain Shahnaz Hussain Zandu Zandu Himalaya
Hair dye	Nourishing hair cleanser After wash hair Conditioner Protein rich hair cleanser Sha-henna Sha-amla Sha-lisma Shama Henna hair pack Nutrisse hair colour mask	Himalaya Himalaya Himalaya Shahnaz Hussain Shahnaz Hussain Shahnaz Hussain Banjara Garnier Garnier
Hair washing	Kuntala powder Aritha powder Shikakai	Green valley Banjara Banjara
Herbal sunscreen	Naturene sunscreen Sunscreen Flawless cream	Naturene Synergie Nature's Way
Infective acne (antibacterial cream)	Antiseptic cream Hide-n-Heal or Shabase	Himalaya (Ayur concepts) Shahnaz Hussain
Moisturiser	Synergie essential moisturiser (oil-free) with almond Synergie nourishing night cream Rich moisturising lotion Moisturising lotion for dry skin.	Synergie Synergie Ayurvedic Concepts Ayurvedic Concepts

Oily skin	Deep cleaning lotion Astringent lotion Shamint (to remove excessive oil) Shazeem (medical soap)	Ayurvedic Concepts Ayurvedic Concepts Shahnaz Hussain Shahnaz Hussain
Pigmentation around eyes	Sha-smooth	Shahnaz Hussain
Pigmentation over cheeks	Sha-white Aqua Bleach	Shahnaz Hussain Shahnaz Hussain
Wrinkling of skin	Anti-wrinkle cream Shalife	Himalaya Shahnaz Hussain

●●

Bibliography

1. *Aroma Therapy* : Gwydion O'Hara
2. *A Treatise on Home Remedies* : Dr. S. Suresh Babu
3. *Body and Beauty Care* : Dr. Neena Khanna
4. *Bhaisajya Ratnavali* : Chowkamba Publication
5. *Green Remedies* : Dr. S. Suresh Babu
6. *Herbal Beauty Care* : Pustak Mahal
7. *Herbal Beauty Clinic* : Paresh Nanda (Pustak Mahal)
8. *Naturally Healthy Hair* : Mary Beath Janssen, Story Books
9. *Natural Hand Cares* : Weing Berg, Story Books
10. *Natural Foot Care* : Tourles; Story Book
11. *Reveal Your Glow* : Donna Rae
12. *Sushruta Samhita*
13. Curr. Sc. 1065-1071 (2003).
14. *Medicinal Plants* : Mac. Donald, London. Chiej, R., 1984,
15. *Rog and Chikitsa* : Hamdard, Delhi.
16. *Handbook of Ayurvedic Medicinal Plants* : Kapoor, L.D.

●●

Home Beauty Clinic

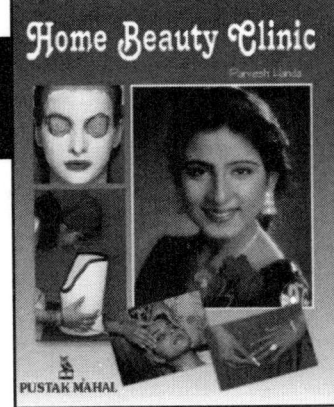

—*Parvesh Handa*

The art of personal beauty care through easily available ingredients is as old a quest as civilisation itself. Today much stress is laid on an attractive and impressive personality, which includes the way of talking, walking, dressing and interacting with others.

Although every woman may not have the fairy-tale looks of Cinderella or the legendary face of Helen of Troy, there is something special and charming in every female. An attractive personality is projected simply by enhancing intrinsic charm and by hiding a person's natural flaws.

Home Beauty Clinic satisfies the various needs of a beauty-conscious woman through modern techniques like facial, massage, make-up, pedicure, manicure, hairstyle, etc. This makes the maintenance of her beauty an everyday affair. Besides, the book also details methods of indigenous preparation of cosmetics, which ensure there are no side effects from synthetic elements.

Big Size • Pages: 128
Price: Rs. 80/- • Postage: Rs. 10/-

Body & Beauty Care

—*Neena Khanna*

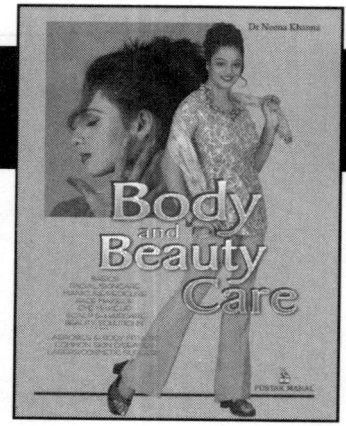

A thing of beauty is a joy for ever. —*Keats*

The image a person projected is of vital importance in career development, opportunity, peer status and ultimate achievement. Poets and artists have long appreciated the crucial role of beauty in human affairs. The latest cosmetic procedures can significantly enhance the appearance of a person.

Body and Beauty Care is primarily intended for the new conscious generation of men and women who groom to look good. Beginning with basic facts about the structure and functioning of the skin, nail, hair and teeth, the book gives the cause and effect of their various problems. It then provides sound advice on the treatment of these problems. A separate chapter deals with modern trends in cosmetic surgery. The book is a must for all those who wish to look good and feel good.

Big Size • Pages: 112
Price: Rs. 80/- • Postage: Rs. 15/-